The Florida Allergy Handbook

UNIVERSITY PRESS OF FLORIDA

Florida A&M University, Tallahassee
Florida Atlantic University, Boca Raton
Florida Gulf Coast University, Ft. Myers
Florida International University, Miami
Florida State University, Tallahassee
New College of Florida, Sarasota
University of Central Florida, Orlando
University of Florida, Gainesville
University of North Florida, Jacksonville
University of South Florida, Tampa
University of West Florida, Pensacola

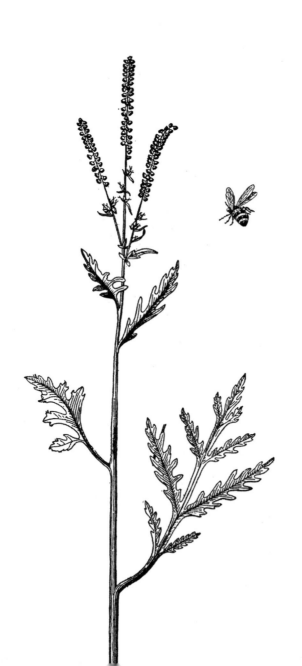

The FLORIDA
Allergy Handbook

Theresa Willingham

University Press of Florida

Gainesville / Tallahassee / Tampa / Boca Raton
Pensacola / Orlando / Miami / Jacksonville / Ft. Myers / Sarasota

17 16 15 14 13 12   6 5 4 3 2 1

Library of Congress Cataloging-in-Publication Data
Willingham, Theresa.
The Florida allergy handbook / Theresa Willingham.
p. cm.
Includes bibliographical references and index.
ISBN 978-0-8130-3746-2 (alk. paper)
1. Allergy—Florida—Handbooks, manuals, etc. I. Title.
RA645.A44W55 2012
362.196'97009759—dc23   2011028205

The University Press of Florida is the scholarly publishing agency for the State
University System of Florida, comprising Florida A&M University, Florida
Atlantic University, Florida Gulf Coast University, Florida International
University, Florida State University, New College of Florida, University of
Central Florida, University of Florida, University of North Florida, University
of South Florida, and University of West Florida.

University Press of Florida
15 Northwest 15th Street
Gainesville, FL 32611-2079
http://www.upf.com

The Florida Allergy Handbook is dedicated to all the family members and friends under whose skin I occasionally got while writing it. Special thanks to my husband, Steve, and my three children, Ellie, Andrea, and Chris, for their patience, love, humor, and indulgence. They're Floridians born and bred, rich in the spirit and character of our remarkable state.

More respect is due the little things that run the world.

E. O. Wilson, *The Creation*

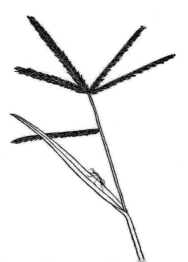

Contents

Preface

The Florida Allergy Handbook provides an in-depth look at common regional allergens and irritants produced by Florida insects, plants, and sea life and examines treatments and preventative measures for ameliorating allergy and injury. It is designed to guide Florida citizens and visitors in safe and enjoyable residential and recreational experiences.

However, this is not a medical book nor is it intended to replace the guidance of professional physicians. It is the result of my own research and experiences and the shared experiences of others and should not be considered a substitute for appropriate care by medical professionals. When in doubt about what to do when you think you or a companion might be having a serious physical reaction to something, call a doctor!

Many thanks to the Florida residents who so generously shared their own experiences and photos within these pages.

Introduction

Gesundheit! Welcome to Florida

Florida is the land of sea and sun. In the Sunshine State, we certainly have an abundance of rays. But we also receive, on average, more than 50 inches of rain annually. That combination of warmth and wet makes for a rich growing medium in which anything can thrive.

What's So Great about Florida?

Besides the great weather, we've got some spectacular landscapes and environments. Florida is home to nearly 3,000 species of plants that live in 80 different natural communities ranging from marine and estuarine environments to hardwood hammocks and pine uplands, all represented across more than 4 million acres of federal conservation land.[1]

We have so much to brag about:

- 1,197 miles of coastline and 663 miles of beaches
- 4,500 islands
- 2,100 square miles of Everglades National Park, comprising the largest mangrove forest and the slowest-moving body of water in the world

- 1,711 miles of rivers
- 1,400 miles of scenic Florida Trail plus hundreds of miles of additional trails
- 161 state parks and hundreds of regional parks
- 700 campgrounds
- 33 first-magnitude springs bubbling out fresh water at a rate of 100 cubic feet per second—more than any other state in the country or any other place in the world

And we've got plants and animals galore! There are an estimated 12,500 insect species in Florida, of which 80 are mosquito species.[2]

There are over 4,100 species of native or naturalized plants in Florida, making it the third most "floristically diverse" state in the United States.[3] There are thousands of species of sea life, over 500 species of birds, and 100 species of mammals.

There are few other places in the country where you can see animals as diverse as alligators and manatees; forests that range from hardwood hammocks of oak and pine to swamps of cypress and mangroves; and warm waters teeming with sea life as tiny as coral polyps, as massive as 800-pound goliath grouper, and everything in between.

Everybody Loves the Sun

And we've got people! According to the U.S. Census, nearly 20 million people actually live here (2009), making Florida the fourth largest state. Another 81 million people visit us annually, a number apparently unaffected by the Deepwater Horizon oil spill disaster in 2010, the most massive oil spill in the history of the Gulf of Mexico. More than 1,000 people move to Florida every day.[4]

Between our 20 million residents and our 81 million tourists, we've got millions of beachgoers, 6 million campers, 1 million boaters, nearly 3 million fresh and saltwater anglers, thousands of scuba divers, snorkelers, hikers, and bikers.[5] And within and around all that great air, land and sea that people are enjoying comes occasional conflict.

The Conflict

Each year, 200,000 jellyfish stings occur in Florida waters.[6] Of our 4,000 plants species, 167 of them produce pollen, and at least 60 of those are known to produce allergic reactions in folks.[7] Several hundred others cause various allergenic responses if touched or eaten. And there are thousands of bug bites and bee stings each year.

The conflict is born of the very nature of nature—which is to make the most of what life gives you, wherever you can find it. Life is nothing if not opportunistic.

South Dakota, for instance—also promoted as the "Sunshine State"—is home to the Badlands, a stark, arid grand canyon of chalklike eroded earth. Nothing would seem able to grow or want to live there. Yet herds of bighorn sheep thrive among the hardscrabble growths of sage and other plants, flowers bloom, and tiny trees take root in the merest hint of shade. Algae and bacteria seem to spring to life in muddy puddles of dew.

So it should come as no surprise that in our peninsular paradise of abundant water, sea breezes, and air so humid you can lean on it, everything and anything that can grow will grow. Even a backyard garden, like every space we try to clear in Florida, is a potential jungle. The more room we try to make for ourselves, the more room we make for everything else and the more we may itch, scratch, sneeze, snuffle, cough, or swell unpleasantly.

That also explains why three of Florida's most crowded metropolitan areas—Orlando, Jacksonville, and Tampa—land squarely among the top "allergy capitals" in the United States, according to the Asthma and Allergy Foundation of America.

How Common Are Allergies Anyway?

Allergies are very common and expensive. According to the American Academy of Allergy, Asthma and Immunology (AAAAI), allergic disease is the fifth leading chronic disease in the United States among all ages and the third most common chronic disease among children under 18 years old. One analysis, says the AAAAI, estimated the cost of allergies at $7.9 billion per year, with $4.5 billion spent on direct care and $3.4 billion on indirect costs, related primarily to lost work productivity.[8]

Here are a few more statistics from the AAAAI:

- Allergic rhinitis is believed to affect about 20 percent of all adults and up to 40 percent of children.
- Approximately 16.7 million physician office visits each year are attributed to allergic rhinitis.
- On any given day, 10,000 U.S. children miss school because of allergic rhinitis, for an annual total of 2 million lost school days.

Just What Is an Allergy?

An allergic reaction is actually a series of events that occur within the immune system upon some sort of physical contact with—inhaling, consuming, or touching—an "antigen"—something the body identifies as dangerous. The immune system is our personal "bodyguard" and consists of specialized cells, proteins, tissues, and organs whose sole job is to keep us healthy and prevent infections caused by antigens.

When triggered, the immune system responds in a couple of different ways, by attacking the antigen with antibodies to capture and consume the invaders and by remembering what triggered the response in the first place, so that the immune system can protect against future encounters.

Immunoglobulin E, or IgE, is the antibody responsible for attacking allergens, and different types of IgE antibodies recognize and attack different types of allergy-producing invaders, ranging from cat dander to oak pollen and bee stings. The exact reasons some people are sensitive to particular things still isn't understood completely, but the reactions in sensitive individuals are similar:

- Chemical "mediators" such as histamine and other chemicals from the mast cells common in the nose, eyes, lungs, and intestines produce the symptoms of an allergic reaction, such as tissue-swelling, sneezing, wheezing, and coughing.

- Newly released mediators recruit other inflammatory cells to that site, resulting in additional inflammation. Those with chronic allergies may suffer excessive swelling, mucus production, and a hyperresponsiveness to the irritating stimuli.

The most severe, and potentially deadly, reaction is anaphylaxis, a whole-body allergic response in which a quick release of large quantities of mediators can cause a sudden and severe drop in blood pressure, a constricted airway and commensurate difficulty breathing, nausea and vomiting, and other symptoms. Estimates of those at risk for anaphylaxis range from a little over 1 percent to 15 percent of the population.[9]

People with a family history of allergies tend to follow suit. If one parent has an allergy, offspring have a 48 percent chance of developing an allergy—70 percent if both parents have allergies.[10]

Types of Allergic Responses

Physical symptoms differ depending on the allergen and where it's released on the body. Types of allergic responses, or diseases, include the following:

- Allergic rhinitis (hay fever)
- Allergic conjunctivitis (pink eye)
- Asthma
- Atopic dermatitis, or allergic skin reactions
- Urticaria (hives)
- Severe allergic reactions to food, latex, medications, and insect stings
- Problems commonly resulting from allergic rhinitis, like sinusitis and ear infections

Allergists and immunologists are the doctors of choice in assessing allergic reactions, and a physician should always be consulted for any severe reactions, like asthma or anaphylaxis, or if you have any questions at all regarding your health.

But generally, allergic reactions are treated in a few standard ways:

- Over-the-counter antihistamines, both topical and oral
- Prescription medications, including inhalers and injectable epinephrine
- Immunotherapy—allergy shots to reduce symptoms

The best treatment, of course, is avoidance, and when it comes to avoiding allergens in Florida, a little education goes a long way.

I'm no stranger to allergies in general. My teenaged son has a wheat sensitivity. In the process of learning how to cope with his condition, first discovered when he was a tot, I learned about many other food allergies and sensitivities and published the results in *The Food Allergy Field Guide: A Lifestyle Manual for Families*.

As a lifelong Florida resident who loves the outdoors, I'm also no stranger to allergies. I've experienced my fair share of sneezing and watery eyes due to hay fever; urticaria swollen hands and feet from some anomalous allergenic contact; hideous poison ivy rashes; blistering ant bites; and recurrent red welts from unfortunate run-ins with sea urchins and Portuguese man-of-war jellyfish. I've been stung, scratched, bitten, and poked by bugs, thorny plants, and sea creatures, gone all-over scratchy from swimmer's itch, and been rendered hoarse from red tide.

Yet I love Florida! I love canoeing, hiking, biking, geocaching, bird watching, and gardening here. I love going to the beach, swimming in the Gulf of Mexico, and combing the beach for shells and shark teeth. I love fishing and boating. I love exploring our parks and preserves. I love watching our wild weather, from the high, bright, and clear crisp blue skies of winter to the lowering purple cumulonimbus clouds of summer.

Presumably all those millions of other residents and visitors love Florida, too, in spite of its bite. But many suffer unnecessarily, and sometimes dangerously, as a result of not being more familiar with some of the dicier aspects of Florida's environment.

So I've written *The Florida Allergy Handbook* to help guide you through visiting and living here safely and comfortably. In the same way that you probably keep a local map nearby when you travel, it's a good idea to know the environmental lay of the land in the Sunshine State. And as you might want to keep a translation guide handy if you go abroad (or to Miami), it's important to know the language of nature here so there are no misunderstandings.

The Florida Allergy Handbook is arranged in four parts:

- Florida (Allergy) Seasons
- Florida Insects
- Florida Plants
- Florida Sea Life

Each section explores allergens and irritants within narrower categories. Reactions that are not technically allergenic are sometimes included for a few reasons:

- They may be encountered commonly enough to provoke concern.
- They may produce reactions very similar to allergens.
- It may be important to be able to distinguish between an irritant and a true allergic reaction.

Covered topics are confined largely to flora and fauna specific to Florida or commonly encountered here. Things like pet allergies and broader categories of food allergies, like those to peanuts, wheat, milk, or eggs, are not covered here because there are numerous resources dedicated to those issues elsewhere. You'll also find internet resources in the appendix and endnotes.

So grab your sunscreen, spritz on the bug spray, light a citronella candle, and keep the antihistamine handy—we're heading into Florida's Great Outdoors!

Part I

Florida Seasons

Hay Fever Season, Mold Season, Oak Pollen Season

Don't let naysayers fool you. Florida definitely has seasons. There's tree pollen season, which generally runs from January to June. Grass pollen season runs from March through October. Ragweed pollen season is in a class all by itself, from July or August until November. And how can we forget mold season during our wonderful hot, humid summers, from June through August—or longer?

Pollen seasons, and the extent of their severity, vary by weather and location. In sensitive individuals, pollen—the tiny particles by which many plants reproduce—can trigger mild to severe allergic responses when inhaled.

Botanist and author Thomas Ogren has developed an allergy rating system for plants known as the Ogren Plant Allergy Scale, or OPALS, which is helpful in identifying the degree to which various plants cause allergies.[1] OPALS ranks plants on a scale from 1, the least allergenic, to 10, the most allergenic, and is being employed by the United States Department of Agriculture (USDA) in their plant documentations. OPALS ratings will be referred to wherever available in subsequent discussions here, noted in parentheses next to plant names.

In his work, Ogren also offers some shorthand clues to identifying plants that are more or less likely to provoke allergies.[2] In general, plants that are less likely to cause allergies include those that have

- showy, perfect flowers, which contain pollen;
- large petals, especially brightly colored ones, and particularly red, orange, blue, or pink flowers, which signify insect as opposed to wind pollination;
- pollen-laden male parts deep inside the flower;
- polygamous plants with separate female flowers, and specifically female-only plants, which are pollen-free;
- lightly aromatic flowers, which attract insects; and
- heavy, sticky pollen that won't travel far on wind.

In contrast, plants most likely to cause allergy problems

- belong to known allergy-causing plant families like the cashew, olive, and spurge families;
- produce a white, sticky sap;
- have long bloom periods (with the exception of orchids);
- bloom even when hard-pruned;
- have tiny (under 30 microns), light, dry pollen or produce pollen in great quantities;
- are male plants;
- have strong fragrances;
- have flowers with exposed stamens or that lack petals or sepals;
- have light, yellow, off-white, or greenish flowers or very tiny flowers; and
- produce spores.

In general, entomophilous, or "insect-pollinated," plants with bright flowers tend to produce heavy pollens that stick around the flowers for better adherence to bees and other insects. They usually don't cause allergy problems.

Anemophilous, or "wind-pollinated," plants, however, disperse high quantities of fine, powdery pollen in an effort to gain fertile distance and improve species diversity. That's great for a tree but not so great for those allergic to its pollen.

What actually causes a pollen allergy is the chemical makeup of the pollen itself. While pine pollen would seem to fit the bill for "bad" pollen, being tiny and produced in such great quantities that it can leave a fine yellowish haze over cars and driveways, its chemical makeup makes it less allergenic than that of oak pollen.[3] The two greatest factors in pollen allergenicity are pollen size and weather. Allergy-causing pollens are typically 20–40 micrometers in diameter, tiny enough to be easily dispersed on windy days or washed out of the air on rainy days.

Not everyone is affected by pollen, of course. Sometimes it just seems that way. But a great many people have no reaction whatsoever. In those better-tuned immune systems, mucus in the nasal passages simply moves pollen particles to the back of the throat to be swallowed or coughed out.

In allergic folks, though, the newly released histamines dilate small blood vessels in the nose. Fluids then escape through the vessel walls, causing the nasal passages to swell and resulting in all too familiar congestion and difficulty in breathing.

Additionally, histamines can also cause itching, irritability, and excess mucus production, otherwise known as sniffling. Other chemical mediators, like prostaglandins and leukotrienes, contribute further to allergy symptoms.

Now that you know the science, let's take a look at the biggest plant-sourced allergy inducers in the Sunshine State.

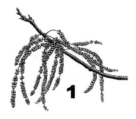

Happy New Year! It's Tree Pollen Season

All things share the same breath—the beast, the tree,
the man . . . the air shares its spirit with all the life it supports.

Chief Seattle

Right around Valentine's Day, people start to notice it—a fine yellowish haze on patio furniture, across the tops of cars, along gutters where it's been washed by sprinklers or the odd winter rain shower. It might be dismissed as dust, but the next day there's a heavier film, and after a few days it coats everything in a relentless powder gone unpleasantly greenish-brown. Seasonal winds can stir things up further.

If you start sneezing and wheezing and go bleary-eyed and snuffly—sure signs of allergic rhinitis—it's easy to blame the stuff for your problems. More than likely, though, it's not the pine pollen being released in copious amounts from tiny male pine cones all around the neighborhood. It's pollen from more allergenic trees like oak, which are releasing their pollen at the same time.

How Tree Pollens Cause Allergies

In a somewhat ironic twist, the less attractive the plant, the greater the chances it will cause allergies. After all, what else has a plain plant got going for it? With no brightly colored flowers, sweet aroma, or cool-looking leaves to appeal to mobile insects, birds, or animals, trees like oaks and pine need to rely on a lightweight, airborne delivery system to get around.

And it's a system that works well. Ragweed pollen has been collected as high as two miles up and four hundred miles out to sea. Tree pollens range far and wide as well. So much for cutting down all the trees in your yard, which, given current climate conditions, you wouldn't want to do anyway. Being allergy-free at the cost of oxygen isn't a very good trade-off.

Understanding Pollen Counts

The amount of pollen grains per cubic meter of air at any given time constitutes the "pollen count" that is often referenced in weather or climate reports. The National Allergy Bureau (NAB), the division of the American Academy of Allergy, Asthma, and Immunology (AAAAI) that collects and reports pollen and mold counts to the public, uses the following scale to describe tree pollen levels:

- Absent 0
- Low 1–14
- Moderate 15–89
- High 90–1,499
- Very high >1,500

Obviously, the higher the pollen count, the greater the chances of allergic reactions in sensitive individuals.

Worst Pollen Producers

Plants produce pollen at times advantageous to their reproductive survival. For trees in Florida, that process usually begins around January and runs through March, coinciding with the High Holy Days of the tourist season. About 82 percent of the pollens during this time of year come from trees, and among those, oak ranks the highest among allergy-producing pollens.[1]

While many often suspect the ubiquitous pine of causing their allergy symptoms, the fact is that pine pollen simply isn't designed in a way that usually causes allergies. That's not to say pine allergies are impossible—primed by all the other trees that may be pollinating around the same time, some people may develop greater than usual sensitivity to pollen of all types, including pine, which nets an OPALS rank of four. The biggest pollen allergy culprits among trees, though, are oaks, birch, maples, mulberry, and Australian pines, which aren't really pine trees at all.

The Mighty Oak (genus *Quercus*) (8)

The single most allergenic tree in Florida is probably the oak tree. There are nineteen species of oak native to Florida.[2] Oaks are members of the beech family, which includes chestnuts and chinquapins.

And they're spectacular trees! Pin oaks (*Quercus palustris*) and turkey oaks (*Quercus laevis*), black oaks (*Quercus velutina*) and laurel oaks (*Quercus laurifolia*), and a dozen other species, with their varying trunks, branches, and leaves and hybridized varieties in between. The live oak (*Quercus virginiana*) is practically synonymous with the South, with its often magnificent spread of gnarled and twisting branches dripping with Spanish moss. Their massive crowns are valuable habitats for birds, insects, and animals, inviting shade for man and beast alike, and a timeless playground for children. Live oak wood, with its natural bends and angles, was used in building ships hundreds of years ago.

In the fall, their acorns rain down noisily on mobile home rooftops and car hoods and crush beneath footfall and tire tread. Many a squirrel ferrying acorns back and forth has met an untimely end standing indecisively in the middle of the road before an oncoming vehicle.

But it's their late winter to early spring activities that can dampen our appreciation of these great trees. Oaks are monoecious—they produce both male and female flowers on the same tree. In oak trees, the female flowers turn into acorns. The male flowers are produced in clusters, or inflorescences, carried in tendril-like growths called catkins.

Each male flower in a catkin consists of a bract (a highly modified leaf), a lobed calyx (sort of like petals), and pollen-producing

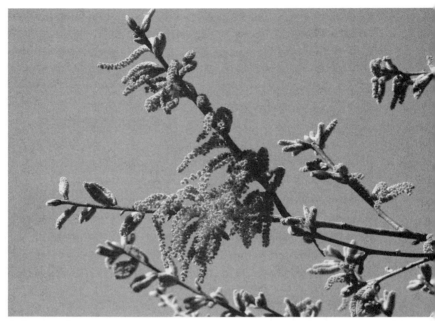

Oak tree catkins. (Photo by Theresa Willingham.)

stamens. Starting around February and continuing through the early summer, catkins release their pollen in copious amounts, causing a commensurate release of histamines in sensitive individuals.

Once the stamens have released their pollen, the spent catkins fall from the tree. If your eyes are red and itchy, you're sneezing and coughing, and your driveway is littered and stained with crumbled little brown catkins, it's a good guess you've got an oak allergy.

Birch (7)

Birch trees aren't nearly as common as oaks here. There are only four or five native species in Florida, the most common being the river birch (*Betula nigra*). But like oaks, birch trees produce catkins, and their pollen causes high reactivity in sensitive people. Birch allergy is also significant for its ability to cause "inhalant-food cross-reactivity" in certain people, or oral allergy syndrome (OAS), also known as pollen food syndrome.

People with OAS have difficulty eating some fresh fruits and vegetables when their seasonal pollen allergies to birch pollen or ragweed are triggered.[3] Up to one-third of people with seasonal allergies may suffer from OAS, which results from a cross-reactivity between seasonal airborne pollen proteins and similar proteins found in some foods.

Australian Pine (*Casuarina equisetifolia*)

Australian pines were brought to Florida years ago to control erosion and act as wind breaks. As equally loathed for their invasiveness as they are loved for the sound the wind makes blowing through their airy branches, Australian pines, which are actually flowering plants and not conifers, produce huge amounts of pollen in the spring.

Australian pines are most common in South Florida. They grow headlong at the rate of five to ten feet per year and have been known to reach heights of thirty feet in just two years.[4] They "bloom" a couple of times a year, once in April and again in September, and are considered a major contributor to pollen season in Florida from December through May and in October and November, particularly in the Tampa Bay area.[5] To add insult to injury, their tiny round, spiky "cones" rival only sand spurs in their assault on bare feet.

Maple

Swamp, or red, maples (*Acer rubrum*) and Florida maples (*Acer saccharum*) are the most common native maple trees, and the females of almost all maple species are among the least allergenic of trees, with an OPALS of 1. But there are dozens of non-native varieties planted as ornamentals, on medians and as landscape trees in neighborhoods and parking lots, and the males of all the maples are highly allergenic, with OPALS of 8 or 9.[6]

Mulberry

Mulberries are among both the most allergenic of trees and the least allergenic. Widely planted as ornamentals, the male mulberry tree is a common cause of allergy problems. The "white" fruitless male mulberry, also known as the "weeping mulberry" (*Morus alba*), native to China where it's grown for feeding silkworms, comes in at the top of the allergy pack, with an OPALS of 10, while the female rates an OPALS of 1. The only native mulberry in Florida is the red mulberry (*Morus rubra*), which can be both monoecious or dioecious, producing copious amounts of pollen as early as March in Florida and continuing well into June.[7]

Melaleuca (*Melaleuca quinquenervia*)

Introduced into Florida a century ago as a soil stabilizer along levees and later as an ornamental, this hardy, almost indestructible exotic with the papery bark had overgrown nearly 500,000 acres of land in South Florida by the early 1990s and eventually established itself on 20 percent of all natural land south of Lake Okeechobee.[8] Also known as the "punk tree," it can produce multiple types of allergies.

The plant flowers from June to November in Florida, and its white bottle brush–like blossoms have a strong and, to many people, a deeply unpleasant odor, which can trigger an allergic response. Its pollen can induce asthma, allergic rhinitis, and allergic conjunctivitis. And essential oils from the plant, commonly sold as tea tree oil, can also cause contact dermatitis.[9]

Other trees known to cause pollen allergy problems include hickory, pecan, walnut, and sycamore.

Diagnosing a Pollen Allergy

The only way to know for sure what type of pollen might be causing problems is to visit an allergist. Symptoms can mimic colds, but when the symptoms linger beyond the usual three days or so, or occur at the same time each year, it's a good idea to see a doctor.

Allergists have a couple of methods for identifying allergy culprits. One is a skin, or scratch, test. Diluted extracts of various kinds of pollen are applied to a scratch or puncture mark and reactions are observed. A positive reaction is usually indicated by a "weal" or a raised red area that develops at the test site.

Blood tests may also be used. The most common blood lab is the radioallergosorbent test (RAST). It's more expensive and not as sensitive as the skin test, and also takes longer—up to several weeks—to yield results.

Treating a Pollen Allergy

The best treatment, of course, is avoidance. In the extreme, that means moving someplace where the plants one is sensitive to don't grow. But that would probably offer only temporary relief, because if allergies are already a problem, chances are good that new sensitivities will develop over time, with repeated exposure to whatever grows in the new environment.

And when you think about it, what's a world without oak trees anyway, with their spreading branches filled with life and light and color? I'll take a sneeze in the shady woods over easy breathing in a sterile house any day. Besides, pollen season is also the best time to be outside enjoying the great weather that caused the pollen in the first place. It's time to garden, hike, bird and wildlife watch, kayak or canoe—all the things that make Florida a great place to live.

Fortunately, there are far less drastic ways to deal with the seasonal problem of tree pollen:

- Stay indoors in the mornings, when outdoor pollen levels are usually the highest.
- Stay indoors when it's sunny and windy, great conditions for trees to release pollen.
- If it's necessary to work (or play) outdoors when allergies are bad, wear a face mask that filters out small particles like pollen.
- Hang out at the beach. (How's that for an excuse to go to the beach? "My allergies are bothering me.") The seashore, with prevailing winds blowing in from the ocean, offers pleasant relief from pollen-laden inland breezes.
- Use air-conditioning—gently. No need to add to climate change with indiscriminate air-conditioning use. But it does help, especially with a good HEPA or other air filter. And change the filter regularly.
- Landscape with (native, if possible) species that do not aggravate allergies, such as crape myrtle, dogwood, fig, fir, palm, or the female cultivars of ash, box elder, cottonwood, maple, palm, poplar, or willow trees.[10]
- Avoid additional irritants like dust, tobacco smoke, and paint fumes, which can aggravate a pollen allergy.

- Dry clothes in an automatic clothes dryer instead of hanging them outside, where pollen can collect on them.
- Shower at night to keep bedding pollen-free.
- Change clothes after coming in from outdoors, and leave shoes outside, so pollen isn't tracked in.
- Bathe pets regularly during pollen season, especially those that come in and out of the house.
- Stay hydrated—with water, not sodas or other sweet or carbonated drinks—to help keep histamines out of your system.

And there are lots of over-the-counter medications that treat seasonal tree pollen allergies, including antihistamines and nasal sprays, as well as prescription medications like corticosteroids.

Separating Treatment Truth from Fiction

Allergies are a common problem, as anyone subject to endless product placement for allergy relief might guess. Exaggerated claims need to be examined for special filters and room air purifiers, for miracle bracelets and magic pills. Consult a local Better Business Bureau or the Federal Trade Commission's Consumer Protection Division for the facts on any health-care product.

Additionally, the Food and Drug Administration and the National Institutes for Health both issue guidance on complementary and alternative medicine. The NIH even has a National Center for Complementary and Alternative Medicine devoted to the study of nontraditional medicine.

Some caveats:

- Small room air purifiers physically can't remove dust and pollen from large rooms (and sometimes even from small rooms) or from the whole house, and they can't protect against viral or bacterial illnesses.
- Electrostatic air cleaners can put unhealthy amounts of ozone into the air, exacerbating allergy and asthma problems.[11]
- Nambudripad's Allergy Elimination Technique (NAET) is a popular new treatment based on the notion that allergies are caused by "energy blockage" that can be diagnosed with

muscle testing and permanently cured with acupuncture or acupressure. There doesn't appear to be any evidence that NAET is effective, although trials have been conducted.

- Magnetic bracelets are touted as a treatment for everything from blocking histamines to stopping arthritis. Generally harmless, there's little evidence that they work, and they may cause allergic responses in those sensitive to the zinc in bracelets.

Allergy Medicines

Use meds carefully, especially in children. Read labels and always consult a doctor before taking any medication. Among the most common treatments are the following:

- Generic loratadine antihistamine or similar 24-hour tablets can be effective for many people and don't cause drowsiness like diphenhydramine can. Antihistamines act by countering the effects of the histamine released by the mast cells. They're usually very effective in relieving sneezing and itching.
- Decongestants act by reducing the swelling and mucus production caused by histamines. They include compounds like ephedrine, phenyl-propanolamine hydrochloride, and pseudoephedrine hydrochloride. However, they can raise blood pressure, increase heart rate, and cause nervousness. And decongestant nasal sprays can become counterproductive if used frequently, creating a "rebound" effect that causes nasal passage swelling instead of relieving it.
- Corticosteroids reduce nasal inflammation and inhibit mucus production. Until recently, they weren't approved for prolonged use because they can cause serious side effects. Today, corticosteroid medication is available as a nasal spray in measured-dose spray bottles, reducing past problems with the medication by enabling it to act only on the nasal passages.
- Cromolyn sodium is basically purified saltwater and is thought to act by preventing mast cells from releasing histamines. It's safe, effective, and doesn't cause drowsiness or other side

effects. Unlike other medicines, though, it must be used for several weeks for a noticeable improvement in symptoms.

Other treatments include combination therapy—using any combination of medicines—and immunotherapy—or allergy shots, which help increase tolerance to a particular pollen.

Immunotherapy involves injecting diluted extracts of pollen under the patient's skin for several weeks, and according to the AAAAI this is successful in 90 percent of patients with seasonal allergic rhinitis and in 70–80 percent with perennial allergic rhinitis. Sublingual immunotherapy trials are also under way to examine the effectiveness of an oral option. Regardless, any medical approach requires consultation with qualified physicians and evaluation of the pros and cons of each.

In Summary

- Tree pollen allergy is common in Florida from January through early summer, depending on the type of tree pollen to which people are sensitive.
- Pollen allergy occurs when sensitive individuals inhale pollens released from allergenic trees like oak or mulberry and the body reacts by releasing histamines to attack the "invaders," causing the classic allergy symptoms of sneezing, coughing, itchy eyes, and general irritability.
- The biggest tree pollen allergy culprits are oaks, maples, mulberry, and Australian pines.
- Pollen allergies are identified via skin prick or RAST blood tests.
- Alternative health claims about magnetic therapy or special air-conditioning filters are often exaggerated and should be evaluated by consumer-safety agencies like the FDA or the NIH.
- Pollen allergy can be alleviated by avoiding the outdoors during high pollen–count periods such as mornings and sunny, windy days, following other pollen-exposure-reduction techniques, taking over-the-counter medications, or consulting with an allergist for more advanced treatments like immunotherapy.

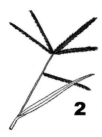

2

Springtime in Paradise

Knowing trees, I understand the meaning of patience.
Knowing grass, I can appreciate persistence.

Hal Borland

Ask folks what natural imagery comes to mind when they think of Florida, and you'll hear of palm trees and sugar sand beaches or maybe swamps and moss-covered oaks. Spend some time driving through our suburban landscapes, though, and you'll soon see that lawns are as much a part of our self-image in Florida as palms and shorelines.

We have dozens of native grasses, with beautiful names like purple love grass, pink muhly grass, and pineywoods dropseed, which are lovely alone or as ornamental landscape elements in a residential yard. But the grasses most people can name are St. Augustine, Bermuda, or Bahia.

Our Love Affair with Lawns

America's nineteenth-century poet laureate Walt Whitman wrote, "I believe a leaf of grass is no less than the journey-work of the stars." Americans would seem to agree.

A few years ago, NASA Ames research scientist Cristina Milesi put together census data, satellite images, and aerial photographs in an effort to estimate how much turfgrass was in the 48 contiguous states. According to her estimates, the United States devotes 128,000 square kilometers, or 40 million acres of land, to lawns.[1] That's more land than we use to grow corn or wheat, potentially making lawns the biggest irrigated crop—to the tune of 238 gallons of water per person per day—in America by surface area.

In Florida, the fourth most populous state, we grow prodigious lawns. In 1992, turfgrass covered more than 4 million acres, 75 percent of which was for home lawns. To feed our green needs, the Florida sod industry grows over 92,000 acres annually.

We Floridians seem to have something of a love-hate relationship with our lawns, alternately fertilizing, watering, mowing, treating for bugs and various diseases, and letting them go to seed and weed. Deed-restricted neighborhoods make headlines every year as they try to crack down on scofflaws with brown lawns, even as drought-stricken communities try to enforce water-use limits. Yet we dump 1.8 billion gallons of increasingly scarce water per day on our lawns and sod farms (58 percent from groundwater sources).[2]

While the money spent on American lawns might be good for the economy—$5 billion in lawn care in 2003 alone—the commensurate pollution from pesticides and mowers isn't particularly good for the environment. And still we mow and edge and treat. And we also sneeze and cough and itch, because grasses are among the most allergenic of plants, affecting 25 percent or more of the U.S. population.[3]

The Grasses

There are more than 1,200 species of grass in North America, over 400 of which grow in Florida.[4] While only a few species cause pollen allergy, grass is second only to ragweed in causing allergic rhinitis—at least out West—and it produces the most severe reactions.[5] In Florida, it gets short shrift next to tree pollen and ragweed, but it's still an important allergen if you're sensitive to it, and a lot of us are.

Grass pollination begins in May and peaks in August. In warm climates like Florida's, it can start much earlier and continue much longer.

As little as twenty grass pollen grains per cubic meter can produce allergic rhinitis in sensitive individuals.[6] Almost all grass allergies are caused by three grass subfamilies:

- Pooideae includes rye, brome, salt grass, orchard grass, and timothy. (Grains like barley and wheat are also in this group, but are self-pollinating and usually don't cause pollen allergies.) Pooideae can also cause commensurate inhalant-food allergy.
- Panacoideae is especially common in the South and includes landscape grasses like Bahia, St. Augustine, and St. Augustine's archenemy (at least in suburbia), crabgrass. Corn, millet, sugarcane, and sorghum are also in this grass group. While sugarcane is usually cut before it flowers, corn and millet are significant allergenic panacoid grasses.
- Chloridoideae includes zoysia and the common recreational turfgrass, Bermuda, which is used extensively on golf courses, sports fields, and parks throughout the South, as well as in some lawns. Zoysia is a common Florida lawn grass.

Behold the Grass Flower

Grasses are pretty remarkable. Over 70 percent of the world's crops are grasses, including rice, wheat, corn, and sugarcane. Relatively "young" in terms of plant evolution, grasses are masters of miniaturization, and they grow from the bottom up—elongated at the base—rather than from the top up, as trees and other plants usually do.

Grasses have the usual plant parts: leaf blades, stems, and, at the appropriate time of year, an inflorescence, or cluster, of flowers that bloom and disperse pollen for reproductive purposes.[7] We don't often think of grass "flowers," but grasses are monocots, whose flower parts typically occur in multiples of three.

In addition to the anther, which, as in most flowering plants, produces the pollen, grasses also have florets and glumes, which are specific to grasses. (They aren't of much significance for those with grass allergies, but *glume* is one of those obscure words that's fun to know!)

Grass Pollen and Allergies

Most grasses are pollinated by wind. Seeing anthers and stigmas hanging all over a lawn signifies that grass has flowered. The actual grass pollen is so tiny it can be carried on the feet of butterflies, and consequently it fits well up inside the human nose. As with tree pollen, grass pollen is regional as well as seasonal, and pollen levels can be affected by temperature, time of day, and rain.

Grass pollens include protein substances, usually enzymes, which are released when the pollen is inhaled. The proteins bind to IgE antibodies and result in the release of histamines and other mediators that cause symptoms of allergic rhinitis, also known as "hay fever."

These grasses typically cause allergies:

- Bermuda grass (*Cynodon* spp.)
- Johnsongrass (*Sorghum halepense*)
- Kentucky bluegrass (*Poa pratensis*)
- Orchard grass (*Dactylis glomerata*)
- Sweet vernal grass (*Anthoxanthum odoratum*)
- Timothy grass, or common timothy (*Phleum pratense*)

Of these, Kentucky bluegrass is the most common sod grass in the country, whereas Bermuda grass, an African import, is the most commonly grown grass in the South. The most common grass in Florida is St. Augustine (*Stenotaphrum secundatum*), followed by Bahia and then Bermuda. While it accounts for only 6 percent of the grass grown in Florida, Bermuda is responsible for 18 percent of grass pollen allergies.[8] It's abundant as a recreational turfgrass on golf courses and playing fields, as well as in suburban lawns, which is pretty remarkable, since it is also considered one of the world's worst weeds.[9]

It earned that distinction with a tough, insistent, and durable nature, thriving in tropical and subtropical climates, adapted to high temperatures, mild winters, and moderate rainfall. In short, Bermuda grass just loves Florida, and Florida loves Bermuda grass. It can even produce seed heads during droughts, and it produces a lot of them: up to 2 million seed heads per pound of grass. That means a lot of pollen, too.

Symptoms of Grass Allergy

Grass can produce allergic rhinitis and contact dermatitis, or "grass intolerance."[10] Grass intolerance, which produces itchy, patchy, or

Table 2.1. Allergy vs. cold symptoms

Allergy	Cold
Runny or stuffy nose, sneezing, wheezing, watery and itchy eyes.	Allergy symptoms plus fever, aches, and pains.
Symptoms begin almost immediately after exposure to allergen(s).	Cold symptoms often develop gradually over the course of several days.
Symptoms last for the duration of allergen exposure and possibly longer. Year-round allergens can produce chronic symptoms.	Symptoms typically clear up within a week. If symptoms last more than a week, visit the doctor for evaluation.

streaky rashes wherever there has been contact with grass, is common among children playing in lawns and fields. I remember getting all itchy after playing in the grass as a child, and I still experience rashes and itching if I sit in certain types of grasses today.

More commonly, though, grass pollen allergy will produce breathing problems due to narrowed air passages and a constant, dry cough with a sore throat. Allergic rhinitis can also produce feelings of itchiness and general discomfort.

Some people find it hard to tell if they're suffering from an allergy or from a cold. Typically, the two are distinguished from one another, as shown in table 2.1.

Additionally, 4 percent of grass pollen allergy sufferers are at risk of developing oral allergy syndrome (OAS), which causes a cross-reactivity in sensitive individuals who eat certain foods, resulting in mouth tingling and itchiness.[11] (More on OAS in chapter 12.)

Ameliorating Grass Pollen Allergy

There's no question that Bermuda grass produces one of the most allergenic of pollens. However, it produces the most extensive pollen when it's stressed and poorly maintained. A lawn that's kept well watered, fertilized, and mowed will produce lower quantities of pollen. According to gardening author Thomas Leo Ogren, a good thick lawn is also a good pollen trap.

"Some years ago," he wrote, "I measured this by sprinkling cedar pollen on different surfaces and then testing to see how much of this pollen became airborne. Of all the surfaces we tested (car roofs, shingles, cement, bricks, different ground cover plants, gravel), none was nearly as effective at capturing incoming pollen as a thick lawn."[12]

Additionally, there are new varieties of Bermuda grass that don't produce any pollen. And the more common St. Augustine grass varieties aren't big allergy producers, either.

That won't help much with wind-blown grass pollens from other lawns, though, especially from leaf blowers, which are the scourge of modern lawn maintenance, not only for their noise and air pollution issues but for the general futility of the idea of blowing leaves and grass around to "tidy" a yard. Mostly, they do a great job of blowing pollen around and add to allergic rhinitis problems.

If work or preference necessitates the use of a leaf blower, wear a mask, and be sure to close windows while a blower is in use to prevent pollen from blowing into your home.

Here are some other tips and tricks for those allergic to grass pollen:

- Consider hiring a lawn service.
- If you must work in the yard yourself, wear a mask.
- Keep grass cut short.
- Use low-pollen ground covers such as Irish moss, bunch grasses, and dichondra.
- Avoid going outside between 5 and 10 am.
- Keep windows in your home and car closed during high pollen seasons.
- Use air conditioners and avoid using window and attic fans, which stir up pollen.
- Dry clothes in an automatic dryer rather than hanging them outside, where pollen can collect on them.

Treatments for Grass Allergy

The best way to treat grass intolerance, or contact dermatitis, is simply to avoid contact with grass. If children show signs of grass intolerance, discourage them from playing in the grass (hard) or encourage them to wear long pants (harder—especially in the summer). Grass intolerance can usually be relieved with an antihistamine or by washing up promptly afterwards.

Grass pollen allergy can be medically treated fairly successfully these days, using a 6 Grass Mix pollen extract, or the extract of the grass that causes the problems, like Bermuda grass pollen extract, depending on skin or blood test results.

A couple of new treatments that show promise in treating grass allergies have made headlines recently. One is a probiotic bacteria drink (*Lactobacillus casei Shirota*) that modifies the immune system's response to grass pollen. The probiotic treatment is still being studied, but early tests have shown significant effectiveness in modulating seasonal allergic rhinitis.[13]

The other is a sublingual grass pollen extract pill called Grazax, which, as of this writing, is available in Europe but not yet in the United States. Grazax has been successful in reducing grass allergy symptoms by nearly 30 percent, and it reduces patients' reliance on antihistamines and steroid allergy treatments.[14] Adverse effects are common, but generally mild, and tend to disappear after a couple of weeks of use. Trials of the medication in the United States began in 2009.

In Summary

- Florida grows over 4 million acres of grass, 6 percent of which consists of highly allergenic Bermuda grass.
- Grass pollen is allergenically volatile: as little as 20 grass pollen grains per cubic meter can produce allergic rhinitis in sensitive individuals.
- Grass is wind-pollinated, its enzyme-laden pollens scattered by a breeze into the air. Once inhaled, these airborne pollens trigger the release of histamines and other mediators in sensitive individuals, producing symptoms of allergic rhinitis, also known as "hay fever."
- Grass can also produce contact dermatitis—hives and rashes—in "grass intolerant" individuals.

- A well-maintained lawn produces little to no pollen and can actually help reduce allergy problems.
- Grass pollen allergy can be ameliorated by taking common-sense precautions like using air-conditioning during high pollen count season, using ground covers instead of grass, and drying clothes in a dryer instead of on a clothes line.
- Though the medical response to allergies usually involves standard immunotherapy treatments, there are some new interventions on the horizon, including a probiotic bacteria drink and the use of Grazax, a sublingual grass pollen extract pill that, shown to be effective in Europe, is currently under study for use in the United States.

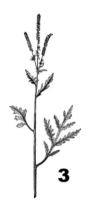

3

Ragweed, the Scourge of Summer and Fall

Solidago, yellow flower of little fame
Now the ragweed gets the best of me, but you always get the
blame.
Solidago, there is sunshine in your name
They all say you're good for nothing, but I love you just the same.

Folk singer Carrie Hamby, "Solidago"

Carrie Hamby waxes eloquent about goldenrod's plight in her song "Solidago," named for goldenrod's Latin identification, *Solidago canadensis*. Indeed, the goldenrod/ragweed issue is probably one of the botanical world's most enduring and unfortunate cases of mistaken identity, as Hamby first learned in a botany class at the University of Florida.

Dr. Loran Anderson revealed the pure silliness of the goldenrod allergy myth one day by pointing out the abundant goldenrod blooms and asking the question: "Why, when a plant has all its pollen conveniently located in these nice clusters, would it need to have pollen floating through the air all the time?"

Then he contrasted it with ragweed, which because it blooms around the same time as goldenrod in most regions gets passed over as the real culprit, and he pointed out the structure of its pollen producing and carrying mechanism. Big difference!

Goldenrod is showy and bright, so it "gets the blame." But ragweed is plain and goes unnoticed while pollen literally explodes from its tiny male inflorescences.

Hamby is right. "Showy" flowers are typically pollinated by insects and are less of an allergy concern than nondescript plants that fly under the landscape radar. Unfortunately, that fact hasn't done much to put the myth of goldenrod allergy to rest.

The Gifts of Goldenrod

About the only things the two plants have in common is that they bloom at the same time, summer through fall, in similar locations ranging from weedy urban areas to open fields. Beyond that, there is little comparison.

Goldenrod produces showy yellow flowers that can paint open fields golden in the fall. Ragweed, as its name suggests, is "raggedy" in appearance, producing small greenish-yellow flowers. Ragweed is the allergy culprit, due to its propensity for releasing up to a billion pollen grains per plant.[1]

Later, Hamby learned about something else that sets the two plants apart and puts goldenrod in unique historical perspective in Florida. While visiting Thomas Edison's winter home in Ft. Myers, she learned about Edison's experiments with goldenrod as a source of rubber. Fascinated, she explored the origins of neoprene coating and naphthalene during the early days of modern chemical engineering and was inspired to write "Solidago," one of her first compositions.

In fact, Edison's experiments with goldenrod, which contains natural latex, produced a twelve-foot-tall plant that yielded 12 percent rubber. The rubber turned out to be resilient and enduring—tires made of the goldenrod compound are still on display at the Edison & Ford Estates museum in Ft. Myers today. But although Edison gave his research to the government before he died, the idea was never developed.[2] Or as Hamby poetically put it,

But the barons of the industry refining oil and gas
then found a petro-chemical for tires that would outlast.

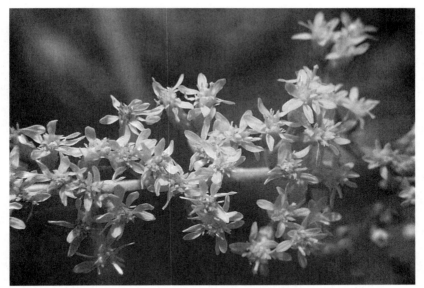

Goldenrod. (Photo by U.S. Fish and Wildlife Commission.)

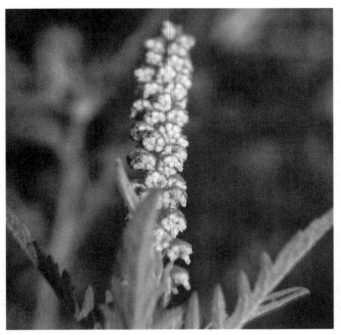

Ragweed. (Photo by U.S. Fish and Wildlife Commission.)

Goldenrod has a long tradition of use medicinally, as a tea, and as a landscape plant.[3] It is the state flower of Kentucky and Nebraska and the state wildflower of South Carolina. "Could we go back to the days before a billion rubber treads?" sings Hamby. "Would we plant our fields in goldenrod, and watch the flowers bloom instead?"

Ragweed Revealed

There are twenty-one species of *Solidago* in Florida, out of about seventy goldenrod species found throughout the eastern United States.[4] This makes it far more abundant than ragweed, of which there are forty-one species worldwide, almost all of which wreak havoc on the human immune system.

The good news is that Florida is home to only four types of ragweed: common, coastal, western, and giant. The bad news is that the common and western ragweed are among the most allergenic to sensitive individuals.

Ragweed is identified scientifically by the ironic Latin name *Ambrosia*, suggesting a culinary delight that doesn't exist. As a matter of fact, even most animals won't eat it, although wild turkeys, quail, and sparrows eat the burrlike ragweed fruit. It did find some redemption among Native Americans, who used the plant to treat nausea and other ailments.[5]

But with ragweed's propensity to cause severe allergic reactions, the healing powers of the plant weren't pursued any further than goldenrod's rubber-making abilities. Of those allergic to plant pollens, 75 percent are allergic to ragweed. It's thought that, overall, 10–20 percent of Americans are allergic to the plant.[6]

Why Ragweed Is So Allergenic

Ragweed is monoecious, meaning it produces both male and female flowers. The male flowers are produced by the thousands in groups of tiny inflorescences, releasing the aforementioned billion pollen grains per plant. A prolific breeder in disturbed areas around the country, ragweed can grow up to fifteen feet tall. It can release a million tons of pollen each year in the United States.[7]

Up North, ragweed begins to flower in early August, peaking in

September and ending in early October, making for a miserable but endurable summer allergy season. Early frosts can shorten the season considerably. In Florida, however, with our balmy tropical weather, ragweed season can begin much earlier, and the plant may even flower year-round, depending on the weather. Add in our great breezes, and ragweed pollen can really get around. It's been found as high as 2 miles up and 400 miles out to sea.[8]

Ragweeds produce pollen more heavily in wet weather, which is sort of a mixed blessing, since increased humidity tends to keep the pollen closer to the ground. But as soon as midmorning dew dries and humidity decreases, or rain clouds move on, pollen quickly becomes airborne.

Because of the long pollinating season, and the size and composition of the pollen grains, ragweed pollen is perfectly designed to throw the human immune system into disarray. And ragweed pollen adds insult to injury by stimulating oral allergy syndrome (OAS) in many people. Ragweed-induced OAS can cause secondary sensitivity to melons, zucchini, and bananas, as well as to chamomile tea and sunflower seeds.[9]

Additionally, ragweed allergy sufferers who ingest honey containing pollen from ragweed or other Compositae plants may have a severe allergic reaction, including anaphylactic shock.

Treating Ragweed Allergy

Besides OAS, ragweed pollen causes all the usual allergic reactions, ranging from mild congestion and annoying hoarseness to more serious asthmatic reactions. There isn't a specific cure for ragweed allergy—only treatments to ameliorate reactions. As with all allergies, the best way to reduce or eliminate ragweed allergy symptoms is to avoid contact with its pollen. That's hard to do with a plant as ubiquitous as ragweed.

The Asthma and Allergy Foundation of America offers the following low-tech solutions:

- Look up the pollen count when planning outdoor excursions. The National Allergy Bureau provides website tracking via www.aaaai.org or by telephone at 800-9-POLLEN.

- Keep windows closed and stay indoors under filtered climate control conditions if possible, utilizing air-conditioning with HEPA filtration.
- Vacation accordingly. You may find relief west of the Rocky Mountains or along the West Coast, where ragweed pollen is less problematic.
- Avoid ragweed habitat, places like ditches, vacant lots, road-sides, riverbanks, and tree lines.
- Drive with car windows closed.
- Remove shoes, shower, and change clothes when returning indoors during high-pollen periods.
- Avoid contact with other known allergens during ragweed season to minimize cross-reactions.
- Use antihistamines and nasal sprays. Newer medications don't cause drowsiness and can control reactions for up to 12 hours.
- Consider immunotherapy, colloquially known as allergy shots. These reduce allergic responses by exposing allergy sufferers to small amounts of the allergen to which they're sensitive, helping them build up immunity.[10]

New Treatments

A couple of new treatments for ragweed allergy are under development. For those who don't respond to antihistamines or traditional immunotherapy, which can take years, an experimental treatment from Dynavax Technologies Corp, based in Berkeley, California, looks promising.

In early 2000, Johns Hopkins Asthma and Allergy Center in Baltimore ran trials with an injection that combined the major ragweed allergen, Amb a 1, with a unique short, synthetic sequence of DNA that stimulates the immune system. Adult volunteers given the shots just once a week for six weeks found that allergy symptoms were reduced for at least one year.[11] Due to the small scale of the trial, long-term safety is still unknown, and more research needs to be done.

Sublingual immunotherapy, developed in 2008, shows equally

good results without shots.[12] It consists of placing minute extracts of allergens under the tongue until tolerance develops. The initial trial consisted of a once-a-day treatment that required the extract to be held under the tongue for one minute and then swallowed. The treatment was started 8–10 weeks prior to ragweed season and continued for up to 10 weeks after ragweed season ended.

Patients in the trial using a higher dose of the drops reported a 90 percent reduction in the need for other antihistamine drops, sprays, or pills during ragweed season. Those using a lower dose reported a 75 percent reduction in the need for other medications. Both groups also reported experiencing a significant reduction in allergy symptoms during ragweed season. Mouth irritation and itching were the only complaints. More studies are in order, but sublingual immunotherapy shows promise.

In Summary

- Goldenrod is often mistaken for ragweed and blamed for causing allergic reactions. Its showy flowers, however, indicate that goldenrod is insect-pollinated, not wind-pollinated like the true allergy culprit: ragweed.
- There are four species of ragweed in Florida: the common, coastal, western, and giant ragweeds. The common and western ragweeds are among the most allergenic to sensitive individuals.
- Although its Latin name is *Ambrosia*, ragweed is not edible except by a few birds and small mammals. It was, however, used medicinally by Native Americans.
- Seventy-five percent of those with plant allergies are allergic to ragweed, and overall, 10–20 percent of Americans are allergic to the plant.
- Ragweed is highly allergenic because it is a prolific breeder, growing up to 15 feet tall with a single plant capable of producing up to a billion grains of pollen. Overall, ragweed releases about a million tons of pollen each year in the United States.

- Ragweed can bloom year-round in Florida.
- Ragweed allergy can cause Oral Allergy Symptom (OAS), producing allergic reactions to certain fruits and vegetables when ragweed is in bloom.
- Ragweed allergy can't be cured, but symptoms can be relieved by (1) staying indoors during high-pollen periods; (2) using HEPA filtration on air conditioners; (3) removing clothing and shoes and showering on coming indoors; (4) using anti-histamines or nasal sprays; and (5) turning to traditional and new immunotherapies.

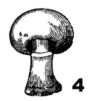

4

A Fungus Among Us

There are spores of fungi everywhere in this world. There are likely to be millions of spores in the room you're in right now, regardless of its general cleanliness. If you're reading this outside, there may be even more spores of many different kinds of fungi. The mere presence of *Stachybotrys* is not a reason for panic.

Thomas J. Volk, mycologist, University of Wisconsin–Lacrosse

The Hogan family moved to Florida from Atlanta when their daughter, Caroline, was a year and a half old. By the time Caroline was three, said her mother, Debbie, she was experiencing hives several times a day. The family thought their little girl had food allergies.

"The doctor told us she had a 'full bucket' and that she was just an allergic kid," said Debbie. "What he meant by full bucket was that she may have had some minor environmental allergies to dust, trees, and molds, but her immune system load was too high. She was surrounded by too many allergens and colds, causing her system to hyperreact to everything, and her 'minor' allergies were turning into major ones."

The doctor directed the family to create a more allergy-free environment for Caroline. "He had us remove all of the allergens from Caroline's sleeping environment, to stop using harsh chemicals in the house, and to wash her clothes with an organic baby detergent from the health food store. I mean we scrubbed our bathtub with baking soda and did our floors with baby shampoo for a long time."

Caroline's health improved somewhat, but she still suffered from daily hives. At about the same time, the Hogan family decided to replace the air ducts in their twenty-year-old Tampa home.

When the repairman cut open the plenum above the garage unit of the air conditioner, said Hogan, "they found mold so thick, and of every color, they could scrape it off with a spoon. It was disgusting."

The company replaced everything, she said, and within three months, Caroline had improved significantly.

"It still seems, though, every year for a month or two in the summertime that she has an environmental allergy that fills her bucket

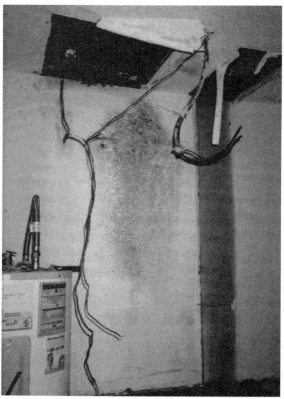

Mold growing around plenum area of Hogan family's air-conditioning unit. (Photo courtesy of Debbie Hogan.)

and we revisit the problems," said Debbie. "But only for a short time, not year-round anymore."

A Brief History of Mold

The phrase "mold and mildew" is actually redundant, since they're one and the same thing. Mildew is simply mold growing, typically, on fabric. And mold is a fungus, one of the five kingdoms of life along with plants, animals, protozoa, and bacteria.

It was seventeenth-century scientist Antony van Leeuwenhoek who declared the kingdom of fungi distinct from that of plants. Among the differences he noted the following:

- Unlike plants, fungi do not produce chlorophyll, and they are unable to make their food. Instead, they release enzymes that break down organic matter into a digestible form from which they can draw nutrients.
- Fungal cells are distinctly different from plant cells, far simpler, tubular in shape and undifferentiated, bearing no roots, stems, leaves, bark, or any of the usual plant features.
- The cell walls of fungi are made of chitin and other polysaccharides, not of cellulose, like plants, or of protein, like animals.
- Fungi reproduce via spores, often produced without any cross-fertilization and usually genetically identical to the parent cell.
- Fungi grow via elongating threads.

It's been estimated that there may be as many as 1.5 million species of fungus, forming a quarter of the Earth's biomass.[1] The different forms of fungi are molds, yeasts, mushrooms, lichens, rusts, and truffles.

Molds are the fungi that typically cause allergic reactions. Although there are 100,000 types of the molds, only about 80 cause health problems for about 10 percent of Americans.[2]

Unfortunately, these few molds cause the majority of indoor air pollution and sickness, with mold colonies, or mycelium, producing millions of microscopic, allergenic spores within days of becoming established.

The Question of Mold Toxicity

We'll touch on this only briefly, since our focus here is specifically allergies. But the question of the true extent of frequently cited inhalational toxicity, more commonly known as "toxic mold syndrome," has been the subject of many studies in recent years.

Molds are known to cause asthma, rhinitis, hypersensitivity pneumonitis, and allergic bronchopulmonary aspergillosis (fungal infection of the lungs) in sensitive individuals, complications often alleviated by immunotherapy and related treatments. But claims beyond those ills that include broader symptoms such as headache, irritability, cognitive impairment, and fatigue, while anecdotally common, remain scientifically unsubstantiated.[3]

In a 2005 study, investigators reviewed the cases of 50 people seeking compensation for toxic mold disease, and in each case they found more compelling explanations for the disorders that were blamed on mold.[4]

That's not to say that mold toxicity doesn't exist. True human mycotoxicosis is well documented, especially in developing nations where direct contact and ingestion of toxic molds and fungi are responsible for food poisoning and even liver cancer.

But molds far more commonly produce the usual allergic responses we've come to know and dislike from our close encounters with trees and grasses.

Mold and Allergies

Mold doesn't ask for much—just a nice damp place to live where it can break down organic matter for dinner. That's pretty much all of Florida.

According to the Florida Department of Health, several types of health problems are caused by molds:

- Allergic symptoms, including congestion, conjunctivitis, coughing, wheezing, skin rashes, shortness of breath, and asthma
- Infections, especially in those with chronic illness or weak immune systems

- Toxic effects that are still under study and mostly occur through ingestion

But inhalation of spores and contact with mold by-products has been implicated in everything from acute pulmonary hemorrhage in infants to Crohn's disease and rheumatoid arthritis. Toxic effects are thought to be caused by exposure to toxins on mold surfaces, rather than mold inside the body.[5]

The most common indoor molds are *Cladosporium, Penicillium, Aspergillus*, and *Alternaria*. These and other molds travel by means of airborne spores that wind up on everything from clothes to pets and inside our noses and respiratory systems.

Mold spores anchor happily and proliferate anywhere they find moisture, including shower curtains, damp walls and roofs, plant pots, urine-soaked areas, and even in standing water. Cellulose-based materials like paper-based products, ceiling tiles, and wood make particularly great mold habitats.

Inhaled mold spores trigger IgE antibodies in sensitive individuals, causing the release of inflammatory agents to mediate the response and the commensurate sneezing, coughing, hoarseness, dry skin, and all the other usual allergic symptoms.

Sensitive individuals may suffer allergy symptoms seasonally or year-round if symptoms are due to indoor molds. When symptoms worsen indoors, especially in damp rooms, mold allergy is a good bet.

Behold the Remarkable Spore

Mold spores are a remarkable invention of nature. Rarely exceeding 100 microns in size, with most less than 20 microns, mold spores sport a variety of distinctive surface features to help them find purchase in their travels.

They have hooks, thorns, spikes, folds, and wrinkles, and each mold produces a uniquely designed spore, with thick, darkly pigmented walls that resist degradation by ultraviolet light and are also able to survive in a wide range of temperatures.

However they differ from one another physically, though, all fungal spores depend on wind and air movement for dispersal, and fungi

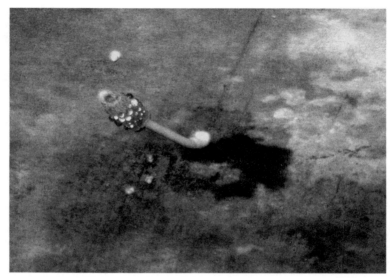

Mushroom growing from hunting cabin ceiling in Dunellon, Florida. (Photo courtesy of Ellie Willingham.)

produce prodigious quantities of spores to improve their chances of reproductive success. Wheat rust fungus, for example, produces 10 billion spores per acre.[6]

Because of their minute size, fungal spores can remain airborne for a long time and travel vast distances quickly. Even on a windless day, a mold spore 20 microns in size can travel seven feet per minute.

In a fascinating test of mold spore agility, Professor C. M. Christensen of the University of Minnesota tested spore dispersal in an office building using distinctively colored mold spores. According to Laurence Molloy in "Pathogenic Fungi," "Five minutes after a culture dish was opened on the first floor, spore of the same fungus were detected on the fourth floor. Five minutes later, spore were falling on the fourth floor in amounts of thousands per square yard."[7]

There's no question that spores in general and mold spores in particular are a tiny, but considerable, force of nature. But there's another potential allergenic trigger in molds that isn't present in other types of plant allergy producers: chitin.

The Chitin Factor

A polysaccharide better known for its role in the exoskeletons of shellfish and insects, chitin is also the single largest component in the cell walls of most molds. According to research led by Dr. Richard Locksley of the University of California in San Francisco, chitin was found to trigger an allergic inflammatory response in the lungs of mice, as well as increased production of a chitin-destroying enzyme made by cells lining our airways.[8]

"Crab asthma" has long plagued those in the shellfish processing industry, drawing particular interest in chitin-allergy research. But applications in mold studies may have more widespread significance to those who suffer mold allergies. Locksley's research suggests that people have innate "chitin-recognition molecules," which cause an immune system response against an allergen or parasite, in part, as a result of the presence of chitin.

In an interesting dichotomy, Locksley draws on the "hygiene hypothesis" to suggest why chitin may be looming large in mold allergies. By sanitizing our homes of dirt and all its commensurate organic material, goes the theory, we've inadvertently rid ourselves of an important ally: bacteria, which are known to reduce chitin. Uninhibited by their natural microbial enemies, molds and chitin-bearing insects are able to run amok in our homes, and their discarded chitin (and other allergy-causing components) are better able to wreak havoc on our immune systems.

Alleviating Mold Allergies

Now that we've dissed housecleaning as being bad for our health, let's revisit it to see how we can properly ameliorate mold problems. And ameliorate it is all we can do, since indoor mold exists in all homes in Florida to some degree.

But there are a few basic practices that can significantly reduce mold in the home. The biggest issue is controlling moisture. To that end, it's important to identify and repair leaks in pipes, minimize condensation from air-conditioning units and duct work, and keep humidity low—which of course, in Florida, typically necessitates running those condensating air-conditioning units. But dehumidifiers and proper ventilation will help keep everything in balance, and so will keeping areas that are frequently wet as clean and dry as possible.[9]

Bleach is an obvious choice for removing mold on nonporous surfaces like countertops, sinks, tubs, toilets, and floors. But moldy porous surfaces, like drywall and carpeting, typically have to be completely removed and replaced.

In a 2001 study for the journal *Aerobiologia,* researchers who sampled 241 rooms in 63 types of buildings found laundry rooms had the highest concentration of mold spore counts, followed by the bathroom and unfinished basements.[10] Basements are not much of an issue in Florida because the water table doesn't leave much space for them. But laundry rooms and bathrooms we've got by the millions. And there are a few things we can easily do to reduce mold in those problem areas and throughout our homes.

Controlling Humidity

A healthy humidity level for mold-sensitive individuals is 45 percent or less, a good trick in a state where relative humidity at least half the year is usually around 60–70 percent (i.e., steamy).[11] Humidity can be measured with a spiffy tool called a hygrometer, which costs between $20 and $30. But some basic rules of thumb can be almost as effective in helping evaluate home humidity.

In the winter, the chief sign that humidity is low is static electricity. Shuffling across a carpet on the way to get the newspaper on a nice winter morning often nets a bright little shock from the door knob that provides as good a jolt as a cup of coffee.

Look out the window on a hot August morning, and a good sign that the humidity is pretty high might be the stream of condensation blocking the view. Lizards and frogs making themselves comfortable in house plants can also be considered omens of dampness. That dampness is exactly what mold loves, and if moisture is collecting on shower curtains, in wall boards, and in plant pots, so is mold.

The best way to keep humidity low would seem to be to set the air conditioner to a low temperature—say 75 degrees—throughout the summer. But that's not an environmentally or economically helpful choice sometimes and, more important, it doesn't guarantee that household humidity will stay below 60 percent anyway, because there's a lot more to humidity than air temperature.

According to the Florida Solar Energy Center, all buildings have leaks.

- Bulk leaks stem from plumbing and rainwater.
- Capillary leaks and diffusion leaks seep from building materials.
- Air transportation leaks occur where water vapor moves through materials due to changes in air pressure.[12]

Additionally, people, animals, cooking, and household water use contribute to indoor moisture.

So the real solution is to control moisture in the home, rather than just temperature alone. There are several ways to help keep things dry and mold-free.

- Use a central air conditioner with a HEPA filtration system.
- Check and clean duct work regularly.
- Make sure there's a working exhaust fan in the bathroom, or open a window when the bathroom is in use.
- Check for and repair plumbing leaks. Leaks can be identified by areas of separating tile, damp wall boards, and mold and mildew along baseboards or door frames.
- Avoid the use of carpeting in bathrooms unless it's removable and washable.
- Clean sinks and bathing areas regularly. An ounce of household bleach to a quart of water makes a reliable cleaning solution.
- Clean refrigerator door gaskets and drip pans regularly.
- Consider using a home dehumidifier.
- Mattresses made of polyurethane and rubber foams are inviting to fungus, so use mattress covers or another kind of mattress.
- Reduce moisture collecting clutter like newspapers and piles of clothes.

- Check water drainage around the home to make sure it flows away from the home's foundation. Keep gutters cleaned out.
- Drain houseplants well or, better yet, keep them on a porch.
- Reduce other outdoor sources of mold—like piles of leaves and mulch and overhanging branches and brush near the home—that can hold moisture and cause mold on outside walls, which can then enter the home as windborne spores.[13]

Diagnosing and Treating Mold Allergies

Mold allergies are diagnosed like other allergies, via patient medical and complaint history, and are usually confirmed by skin tests exposing the patient to extracts of various fungi. As with most allergies, the main treatment is avoidance of the allergen, most likely spores, in this case, and possibly chitin. As with most allergens, this avoidance can be difficult. Spores are just hard to duck, and avoiding chitin is like avoiding dust.

There are some safe practices that may help, however.

- Wear a dust mask when gardening, cleaning, or working in areas where you are apt to be exposed to mold.
- Stay inside (a dry, low-humidity, HEPA-filtered home) during periods of high mold spore concentration, which can be tracked via the American Academy of Allergy, Asthma and Immunology's National Allergy Bureau alert system.
- Use over-the-counter antihistamines and decongestants to relieve symptoms.
- Consider immunotherapy treatment—allergy shots—to improve resistance to the components of mold that trigger allergic responses.

In Summary

- Mold and mildew are the same thing. Mildew is simply mold growing on fabric surfaces.
- Mold is a fungus, one of the five kingdoms of life, and among the most abundant living things on earth, making up a quarter of the earth's biomass.

- Chitin, the same substance that comprises the hard exoskeleton of many insects, is also present in fungal cell walls and may be a component of mold allergy.
- Molds like damp environments and reproduce via minute and sturdy potentially allergenic spores that can travel seven feet per minute and are resistant to extreme temperatures and ultraviolet light.
- Of the more than 100,000 molds known, only about 80 cause health problems for the 10 percent of Americans sensitive to molds. The most common indoor molds are *Cladosporium*, *Penicillium*, *Aspergillus*, and *Alternaria*.
- While mold spores are known to cause asthma, rhinitis, hypersensitivity pneumonitis, and allergic bronchopulmonary aspergillosis in sensitive individuals, the true extent of "mold toxicity" remains under investigation.
- Mold allergy can be alleviated by reducing humidity in and around the home with dehumidifiers and proper ventilation.
- The highest concentration of mold spores in a home usually occur in the laundry room and bathroom, so these rooms should be kept clean and dry at all times.
- Mold allergies are diagnosed and treated like other allergies; treatments include avoidance, use of over-the-counter medications, and immunotherapy.

Part II

What's Bugging You?

People need insects to survive, but insects do not need us.

E. O. Wilson, *The Creation*

Some may take issue with biologist E. O. Wilson's assessment of the insect world. But the fact is that while Florida is quite literally abuzz with bugs, many of which seem to view us as a convenient buffet, most would do quite well without us. It's a bug-eat-bug world, and problems between humans and insects usually occur when we blunder unprepared into an environment better suited for them than for us.

It's hard to take an insect census, but according to a wonderful little article called "Precinctive Insect Species in Florida," authors J. H. Frank and E. D. McCoy of the University of Florida estimate that there are about 12,500 insect species in the state, accounting for millions upon millions of individual insects.[1] (Just for perspective, there are thought to be 900,000 types of known insect species in the world, representing 80 percent of the Earth's animal species!)[2]

We have over 3,000 species of bees, wasps, and ants, 100 species of horseflies and deerflies, 80 species of mosquitoes, 25 species of cockroaches, and similarly impressive collections of spiders, beetles, and caterpillars.

Insects, bugs (they're not the same), spiders, and other arthropods are everywhere in Florida, trilling, ratcheting, whirring, fluttering, whizzing, digging, burrowing, drilling, pollinating, killing, eating, drinking, and making more of themselves. Many are beautiful, or at least striking in appearance. Many are amazing in habits and lifestyles. A lot of them bite. Most are harmless. Some are deadly. And some cause allergies.

Of the millions of people bitten or stung annually by arthropods, that class of creatures including insects and arachnids, about 25,000 individuals suffer severe injuries, and about 30 die of those injuries.[3] To put that in perspective, the odds of getting bitten by a bug in Florida are far higher than your chances of getting struck by lightning here.

But the odds that you'll suffer a severe reaction to an insect bite or sting are far lower than a lightning strike, although higher than a shark attack. Given how a lot of people feel about insects in general, many would view that as good news and go play golf in a thunderstorm or even take their chances swimming at dusk. (Both are bad ideas, by the way.)

Insect Venom

Still, we do have a lot insects, and many of them produce some type of venom. About 15 to 20 different types of Florida arthropods produce venom sufficiently toxic to produce everything from skin reactions to respiratory problems and potentially anaphylaxis.

Insect venoms typically produce any of four types of physiological reactions:

- Blistering, from the vesicating (blister-causing) toxins produced by blister beetles, some caterpillars, and millipedes
- Central nervous system reactions from the neurotoxins produced by black and brown widow spiders, certain scorpions and ticks, Hymenoptera (bees, wasps, and ants), and wheel bugs
- Tissue destruction from the cytolytic (cell destroying) and haemolytic (red blood cell destroying) toxins of Hymenoptera, fire ants, some scorpions, mites, chiggers, wheel bugs, and the brown recluse spider
- Blood clotting problems due to the hemorrhagic (profuse bleeding) effects of the toxins in the bites of lice, fleas, ticks, mites, true bugs, and biting flies[4]

These various responses to insect bites are not allergenic in nature, involving the immune system, but rather the immediate reactions to insect toxins. According to the University of Florida IFAS, "Allergic reactions to stings or bites are when something happens to a part of the body other than the immediately affected area."

The swelling you have at the site of a bee sting is a localized response to the toxicity of the venom. Not being able to breathe within a few minutes of a bite is a systemic allergic reaction. Up to 3 percent of individuals may be at risk of severe allergic reaction (known as anaphylaxis) to insect stings.[5]

Allergic Reactions

Allergic reactions occur when immune systems overreact to the venom in an insect sting, usually after someone has been sensitized to the insect venom from a previous sting. Upon a subsequent sting, the now oversensitized immune system releases histamines into the bloodstream to combat the venom. The histamines dilate blood capillaries, causing warmth and redness on the skin. Swelling around the sting site, hives, and itching result from fluid escaping from the now more permeable capillaries into surrounding tissue areas.

Severe reactions that progress to anaphylactic shock occur when the swelling extends to the tissues of the throat causing difficulty breathing and, potentially, death. A study of 641 deaths due to yellow jackets, bees, and wasps reported respiratory congestion accounted for more than half the fatalities.[6]

Dermatitis

Among the milder, more common reactions to many insect encounters is some form of dermatitis. There are two types of dermatitis that can occur from contact with insects, plants, and other potential skin irritants: irritant contact dermatitis or allergic contact dermatitis. Insects can cause either or both.

Irritant contact dermatitis accounts for 80 percent of all contact dermatitis cases.[7] Irritant dermatitis is chemically induced, with symptoms typically more painful than itchy and occurring within a few minutes to several hours after contact.

Allergic contact dermatitis is an immune system response that can be triggered after one or two exposures to a substance to which an individual is sensitive. Reactions ranging from itching to rashes can occur within 4 to 24 hours of exposure, although in the elderly, reactions can be delayed for up to four days.

In *Stinging or Venomous Insects*, P. G. Koehler and F. M. Oi classify allergic reactions to stings as follows.

Slight   Mild inflammation, welts, itching, malaise, anxiety.

General   The above, plus two or more of the following: swelling, wheezing, abdominal pain, nausea, or vomiting.

Severe   Any of the above plus two or more of the following: difficulty in breathing, difficulty in swallowing, hoarseness, confusion, or feeling of impending disaster.

Shock   Any of the above plus two or more of the following: cyanosis, drop in blood pressure, collapse, unconsciousness, incontinence.

The latter two reactions, of course, most people want to avoid. And the best way to avoid problems with Florida insects is to be informed, proactive, and prepared.

So douse yourself with some DEET and pull on the mosquito netting. We're going in for a closer look!

5

Beeware of Hymenoptera, Part I

Bees and Wasps

If a bee stings you once, it's the bee's fault;
if a bee stings you twice, it's your own damn fault.

A Dictionary of American Proverbs, edited by Wolfgang Mieder

The good news is that insects don't purposely seek out people to sting. The bad news is that while insects rarely attack without provocation, humans stumble into harm's way all the time, sometimes with deadly consequences.

In 2002, an 83-year-old Odessa, Florida, man was driving his riding mower through a wooded area near his driveway when vibrations from his mower evidently disturbed an underground nest of yellowjackets. His wife found him dead in their yard. Entomologists arriving at the scene 20 minutes later found wasps "still swarming in a tornado-like fashion around the lawnmower." They estimated that the underground nest may have been home to 10,000 yellowjackets.[1]

That's an extreme case, of course, and the man's death was due more to the overwhelming toxicity of so many wasp stings, known as mass envenomation, than to any allergic reaction. According to University of Florida researchers, an adult man would have to be stung 1,500 times to suffer fatal consequences. Most people stung by yellowjackets and other wasps and bees have mild reactions, typically redness, swelling at the site of the sting, itching, and some pain.

Of the stinging insects in Florida that most people probably want to avoid, those of the order Hymenoptera, which includes yellowjackets, are among the most problematic. The Hymenoptera group includes the following insects:

- Yellowjackets and hornets (*Vespula* and *Dolichovespula spp.*)
- Honeybees (*Apis mellifera sp.*)
- Paper wasps (subfamily Polistinae)
- Fire ants (genus *Solenopsis*)[2]

Hymenoptera have venom so strong that, in very sensitive individuals, stings can result in death in less than one hour.[3]

Before retreating into the house with a can of wasp and hornet spray, though, let's step back and take a realistic look at these fascinating insects and learn how to give them the wide berth they deserve to preserve the safety we need.

Hymenoptera Up Close and Personal

Hymenoptera are a diverse group of insects. Estimates of the number of species in the order vary between 3,000 and 6,000. One thousand species of Hymenoptera have been identified at the Archbold Biological Station in Lake Placid alone. Insects of this order are characterized mainly by their two pairs of transparent wings, of which the forewings are much larger than the hind, a trait seen more readily in lab-mounted specimens than quickly moving live ones, and ovipositors that can double as stingers.[4]

In many species the ovipositor is just that, an egg-laying device. Sawflies, horntails, and wood wasps may resemble their more aggressive cousins, but they neither sting nor bite. Some, however, like the sawflies, are responsible for significant forestry damage as a result of using their wood-boring ovipositor to deposit destructive larvae in trees.

Fortunately, even among the stinging Hymenoptera, there's something of an honor code: the stray single bee or wasp will seldom sting.

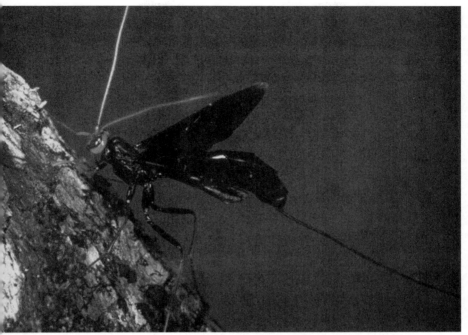

Ichneumonid wasp. (Photo courtesy of University of Georgia Archive, University of Georgia, Bugwood.org. This work is licensed under a Creative Commons Attribution 3.0 License.)

On their own, bees and wasps use their stingers to disable prey, and there's rarely any mistaking a lumbering human for a jumping spider or cricket. And solitary Hymenoptera like mud daubers, which live alone and make links of individual mud cells for their larvae, won't even attack when their nests are being removed.

It's mostly when people get too close to the nests of highly social Hymenoptera like honeybees, where larvae and adults are present together, that social protectiveness, with the accompanying phero-mones, kicks in. So let's start there.

Bees (family Apidae)—Allergy Potential: Moderate to High

The chances of being stung by a bee are relatively slight, and the po-tential for bee venom allergy is moderate for most people, although higher for those with occupational exposure, like beekeepers, or those who are very sensitive to bee venom.

Between 15 and 25 percent of the population can become sensitized to Hymenoptera venoms, with numbers higher in rural areas where there is more contact with bees and wasps. Severe allergic reactions have been estimated to occur in up to 5 percent of the population.[5] According to one report, though, the threat of truly deadly allergic reactions may be overstated in much literature, given the historical lack of supportive epidemiological studies.[6]

Dr. Howard S. Rubenstein, of the Harvard University Allergy Clinic, suggests there is an important difference between "frightening systemic reactions," which can and do occur, and "life-threatening reactions," for which there appears to be little to no evidence. Bee sting deaths may result from a number of mechanisms, but the most common appears to be atherosclerosis (plaque in the arteries), not allergy. Anaphylaxis, he asserts, remains an extremely rare occurrence.[7]

Be that as it may, stings hurt and will no doubt produce some sort of reaction, from a painful localized response to a possibly frightening systemic one. The venom from both honeybees and bumble bees (which rarely sting) is cross-reactive, meaning exposure to either can stimulate an allergic response in sensitive individuals.[8] Chemistry buffs might enjoy learning that bee venom is a complex, mostly enzymatic, mixture of peptides and glucoproteins.[9] Most folks, though, just want to keep a low profile when it comes to bees.

The Scoop on Bees

There are 20,000 species of bees worldwide, 4,000 in the United States.[10] Six families of bees take up residence in Florida, and while they're among the stinging members of Hymenoptera that can be dangerous to allergic individuals, we quite literally can't live without them.

They're vital for the successful pollination of citrus and other fruit and vegetable crops, as well as the reproductive health of countless native plants.[11] Unfortunately, in recent years, bees nationwide have suffered serious setbacks from colony collapse disorder and other diseases.

Bees are typically thick-set, short-bodied insects, often "hairy" in appearance. The bees people are most likely to encounter in their daily Florida lives are honeybees, halictid bees, leaf cutter bees, and the big bumble bees and carpenter bees. All of them sting, but the honeybee is the only one that almost always leaves its autonomously pumping stinger in the victim.

In and of themselves, bees are generally not aggressive. Beekeeping is an admirable and enjoyable hobby. Bees droning from flower to flower are a marvel to watch, and their reputation for being industrious is well earned. They keep their hives clean and tend to their larval children and their queen with devotion, even providing collective cooling for their nest by beating their wings in concert near the entrance.

Our "Beeline" highway in eastern Florida, between Orlando and Cocoa, is a man-made tribute to their efficient transportation methods that always lead them back to their nests no matter how far they've traveled. They use pheromones, a chemical language, to lay down special bee paths, communicate the location of food, and signal alarm.

The alarm pheromone is the one that causes problems for people and pets. When sufficiently disturbed, bees will exude an alarm "scent"—a pheromone—that triggers other bees to come to the aid of the hive. This scent is heavily deposited around the stinger and venom sack, so that when a bee stings, it's also still signaling other bees where to attack. It's an admirable defense system unless one is on the receiving end, especially if bee venom allergy is an issue.

Bumble Bees and Carpenter Bees

Bumble bees and carpenter bees are similar in appearance, spectacularly big, and highly social. They're also big on conflict avoidance. Bumble bees are easy to recognize from the corbicula, or "pollen basket," usually visible on a back leg. Honeybees have this feature, too, but the bumble bee dwarfs them, ranging from ¾ inch to 1½ inches in size.

The old wives' tale that bumble bees aren't aerodynamically built

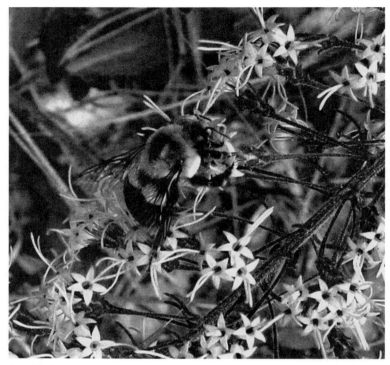

Bumble bee on pentas. (Photo by Theresa Willingham.)

to fly is just that: an old wives' tale, probably brought about by the bumble bee's appearance, with its large head and body and small wings. Obviously, the bee flies quite well.

The carpenter bee is similar in appearance to the bumble bee but lacks hair on its abdomen, giving it a shinier appearance. Additionally, its head is squarer and proportionally larger.

Carpenter bees, as their name suggests, tend toward woodworking, boring holes and tunnels in trees and deck work. Like the bumble bee, they're not aggressive. But both will sting if provoked.

Having once stuck my hand into a clothespin bag where it met up with a carpenter bee, I can tell you the sting hurts. But the bee doesn't usually hang around for more, and this one retreated as quickly as I did.

Halictid Bees and Leaf Cutter Bees

Also known as "sweat" bees and green metallic bees, halictids are abundant, solitary little green bees with the off-putting habit of landing on sweaty people to lap up their salt-laden sweat. They don't seem to do this very much in Florida, where it's thought that sufficient salt and related mineral components are plentiful for them in our coastal environment.[12]

Halictid bees are common in disturbed areas, and usually nest in deep burrows underground. They may sting when brushed away, but aren't considered a significant threat to people.

Leaf cutter bees are about the size of honeybees, stout-bodied, black, and also solitary. They cut out neat sections of leaves with which to build a remarkable cigar-shaped nest composed of individual cells, each of which contains an egg.

They're also placid bees and will sting only when handled—such as when a gardener becomes annoyed at the chunks they've taken

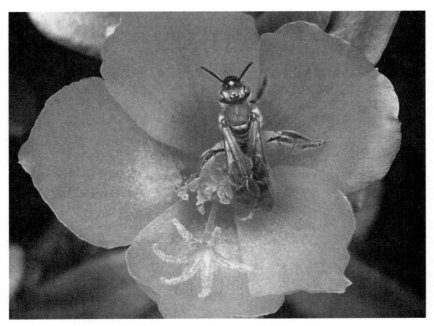

Halictid bee on purslane. (Photo by Andrea Willingham.)

out of an ornamental plant and try to swat one away. If it's any solace, the damage is only aesthetic and the bees don't harm the plant.

European versus Africanized Honeybees

Of the bee families, honeybees make the news most often, especially the much-dreaded Africanized honeybee, which often carries the appellation "killer bee." All honeybees are imports, the first ones in America coming ashore with the pilgrims.[13] But the Africanized honeybee, or *A.m. scutellata*, is distinct from the more peaceful and cooperative European honeybee, *Apis mellifera,* with which a well-intentioned Brazilian scientist, Dr. Warwick Kerr, attempted to breed them in the mid-1950s.

Unfortunately, the aggressive African ("African" and "Africanized" are used interchangeably) honeybees proved deeply uncooperative, swarmed before their quarantine period ended, and have been spreading throughout South America and the southern United States, occasionally taking down livestock, pets, and people for the past fifty years.

The African honeybee isn't significantly different from the European honeybee in habit or appearance. It's a little smaller, but its most distinguishing characteristic is its extreme defensiveness. Where an accidental intrusion on a European honeybee hive in the woods might net a painful response from ten or so bees, a similarly unintentional blunder into *A.m. scutellata* territory can result in a potentially deadly attack by over 1,000 Africanized bees.[14] They also claim a much larger personal space than European honeybees and take offense much more quickly.

Consequently, the African honeybee's threat lies less in the potency of its venom—which is identical to that of the European honeybee and probably delivered in a smaller dose, due to its smaller size—than in the sheer quantity of stings a horde of angry bees can deliver.

Treating Bee Stings

The honeybee is the only stinging Hymenoptera that has a special-delivery venom package: its stinger detaches into the victim where

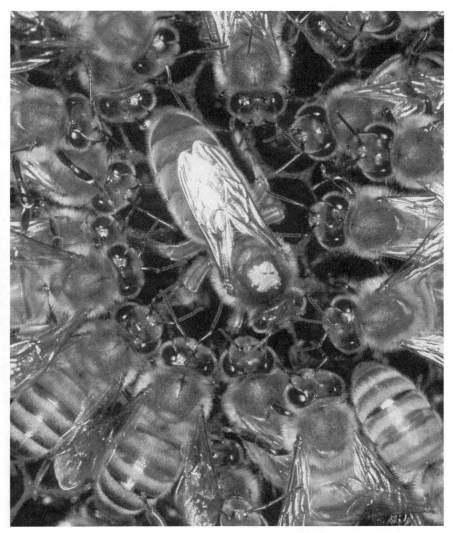

Closeup of Africanized honeybees (AHBs) surrounding a European honeybee (EHB) queen, marked with a pink dot for identification. Since AHBs arrived in Texas in 1990, they've mated with EHBs and spread throughout the Southwest. But rather than commingling, AHBs tend to replace EHBs, partly because EHB queen bees mate disproportionately with African drones. (Photo by Scott Bauer, USDA Agricultural Research Service, Bugwood.org. This work is licensed under a Creative Commons Attribution 3.0 License.)

it continues to pump venom by itself. This ultimately kills the bee, since it has just torn off a vital body part.

Of more immediate concern, after being stung, is evacuating from the area where the sting has occurred, in the event that there's been an accidental encroachment on a hive. After getting out of harm's way, the next thing to do is to quickly remove the venom-filled stinger.

Conventional wisdom has always dictated removing the stinger with some sort of straight edge to prevent squeezing more venom into the wound. However, a rather interesting University of California, Riverside, study suggests that speed is of greater essence than any well-intentioned protocol.

"The method of removal is irrelevant, but even slight delays in removal caused by concerns over performing it correctly (or getting out a knife blade or credit card) are likely to increase the dose of venom received. The advice should be changed to simply emphasize that the sting should be removed, and as quickly as possible."[15]

"Quickly" is the operative word, since most of the venom from the stinger can be injected within twenty seconds.

For treating localized reactions, like pain and swelling at the site of the sting, consider these remedies.

- Apply an ammonia-based sting treatment. This remedy works quickly to break down venom protein but is only effective within 15 minutes of a sting.
- Apply ice. Ice is a quick and useful neutralizer and soother and in most cases reduces the reaction considerably.
- Over-the-counter oral antihistamines reduce reactions further and can be taken for a couple of days after the sting.
- Hydrocortisone creams can also be helpful.

For generalized allergic reactions, a visit to the doctor may be in order. Treatments will vary with severity and can include the following:

- Oral prescription antihistamines
- Injected chlorpheniramine (an antihistamine)
- Intramuscular chlorpheniramine and hydrocortisone
- Inhaled asthma treatments.

Individuals who suffer generalized allergic reactions may want to consider immunotherapy for protection against future stings. Venom skin tests can help verify the specifics of the venom allergy, and then tailored immunotherapy over a period of years can provide long-term protection.[16]

The best treatment for bee stings, though, is avoiding them in the first place.

Bee Control and Injury Prevention

Bees, for better and for worse, are attracted to many of the same bright and beautiful blossoms Floridians enjoy. And they tend to nest exactly where they're most likely to be disturbed by those who, with the exception of bears and beekeepers, are least likely to want to disturb them. They'll build hives in everything from small empty buckets and boxes to old tires, abandoned or neglected cars, lumber piles, sheds, garages, beneath decks, and under buildings. While they prefer building hives in tree hollows and other sheltered locations, honeybees will even build a nest in the open, if needed.

The corollary of our shared affinity for flowers, of course, is that if we insist on having flower gardens, we must be prepared to coexist with the bees that help make the gardens beautiful. Conversely, one way to help minimize bee activity in a yard is to try selecting plants that don't attract bees. These include ornamental grasses, plants that draw butterflies and hummingbirds with long tubular type flowers, and ground covers with tiny flowers, like sunshine mimosa or Asiatic jasmine. Of course, one can't stop neighbors from enjoying their flowers, and bees don't respect property lines, so caution always has to be exercised with respect to bee nesting behavior.

A useful book produced by the University of Florida Cooperative Extension Service includes this wonderful piece of advice: "If a bee swarm is undesirable in trees, shrubbery, or buildings, you may wish to contact a beekeeper, county agent, or pest control company to remove or kill the bees."[17]

It's hard to imagine many instances where a bee swarm would be desirable in a building, but the point is well taken. If buzzing is evident upon entering an outbuilding or when nearing a portion of yard, forest, or field, look for bee traffic that might indicate a hive, keep clear, and call in professional help, if needed.

Similarly, examine work areas before using noisy power equipment in a yard or near potential bee sites, because vibrating equipment and bees don't mix. Caution is also important when penning livestock or when outdoors with pets, especially dogs who, upon disturbing a nest, may understandably "make a beeline" back to an owner, followed by a swarm of angry bees. It should probably go without saying that it's not a good idea to purposely disturb a swarm or colony of bees or hang around with people who do.

Regular weekly inspection of the home throughout the spring and summer and, periodically, year-round, as well as preventative bee-proofing, go a long way toward maintaining a safe zone around house and yard. Here's how to practice good bee-proofing:

- Clear away potential nesting sites, such as empty containers and wood piles.
- Seal any openings greater than one-eighth of an inch in walls, around plumbing, or around window areas of sheds or other outbuildings.
- Install screen or hardware cloth over rain spouts, vents, tree cavities, fence posts, utility boxes, or any other inviting openings into houses or buildings.[18]

Outdoor Safety

Bees are most active in the spring and summer months, the same time Floridians are enjoying the great outdoors. But there are some basic outdoor recreational safety precautions that can help:

- Avoid working near flowering ornamentals when bees and wasps are collecting nectar.
- Wear shoes when outdoors.
- Cover sodas, lemonades, and other sweetened drinks or fruit being enjoyed outdoors. Bees and wasps tend to slip inside an unguarded soda can and can deliver an unwelcome surprise at the next sip.
- Don't swat at bees. It's generally useless and tends to provoke the trouble that one is trying to avoid.

Hikers, joggers, fishermen, and nature watchers who keep to marked and well-maintained trails and recreational areas in Florida parks and preserves will seldom encounter a beehive. On the other hand, hunters and others who stray into unmarked and undisturbed natural areas have increased chances of getting in harm's way. Here are some tips for ensuring maximum safety in parks and preserves:

- If a hive is encountered near a well-used trail, give it a wide berth and notify park personnel.
- Wear light-colored clothing, including socks, shoes, and hat. Bees will defend their hives against what appear to be natural predators like bears and tend to target dark objects. Bees also see red as black, so fluorescent orange safety clothing is a good option for hunters.
- Avoid wearing perfumes, strongly scented shampoos, lotions, or oils or using citrus aromas, all of which may attract or provoke honeybees, especially Africanized honeybees.
- Keep escape routes in mind when outdoors. Retreat is the order of the day with bees. If stung, move away from the area quickly and seek protective shelter to remove stingers and proceed with treatments.

Wasps and Hornets (family Vespidae): Allergy Potential— Moderate to High

The allergy potential from wasp stings is similar to that of bees, although bee and wasp venoms contain some distinctly different chemical properties.[19] But those allergic to wasp venom are only rarely also allergic to bee venom.

As with bees, reactions can be generalized or local. While wasp stings may not occur as often as bee stings, sensitization to wasp venom requires only a few stings and can occur after only a single sting.[20]

Wasps

While bees, despite the occasional sting, are considered admirably industrious—being "busy as a bee" is a compliment—wasps and hornets evoke very different images. Even their names sound sharp and threatening, and they've been invoked in language and literature throughout history to denote dangerous territory and cautionary conduct.

Pope Paul VI warned, "Anger is as a stone cast into a wasp's nest."

"When you are in politics, you are in a wasp's nest with a short shirt-tail," said Mark Twain.

And then there's this rich visual from French playwright Sébastien-Roch Nicolas De Chamfort (1741–94): "Scandal is an importunate wasp, against which we must make no movement unless we are quite sure that we can kill it; otherwise, it will return to the attack more furious than ever." And warnings against "stirring up a hornets' nest" have abounded in American idiom since the pilgrims.

So it's no wonder many of us duck and dodge when a wasp drones by with dangling legs or a hornet buzzes near. But like all the rest of Hymenoptera, a little knowledge goes a long way toward understanding insect behavior and staying safe.

Hunter Wasps (family Sphecidae)

The hunters are the biggest and most eye-catching of the wasps. Principal among them is the cicada killer, or giant ground hornet, and at up to two inches long, it's one of the largest and most spectacular wasps in Florida. Cicada killers do just as their name implies: to feed their larval young, they prey on cicadas, those trilling insects that chorus loudly throughout summer evenings.

Conversely, and appearances to the contrary, they are also among the least threatening insects in the wasp group. The females of the most common Florida species of cicada killer, *Sphecius speciosus*, are the only ones that sting, although they're better known for their amazing trenching ability. They dig burrows up to a foot or more deep, with cells and branching tunnels in which they lay their eggs, along with a cicada meal for the young to eat when they hatch.[21]

Cicadas are physically harmless to people, but can decimate crops. They're large insects—hence the size of the wasp that preys on them. And because cicadas can be so destructive, cicada killers are considered a beneficial insect with respect to controlling an agricultural pest.

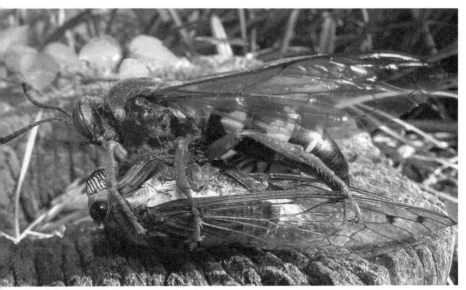

Cicada killer with cicada. (Photo by H. A. "Joe" Pase III, CF Entomologist, Texas Forest Service, Forest Pest Management. Used with permission.)

While the female may sting if disturbed and the sting is said to be very painful (it's a big wasp!), they're solitary insects and, as such, not quick to attack, nor are their stings known to be allergy triggers. The males are more aggressive and have the bothersome habit of dive-bombing people in their territory, but they don't sting, relying, as do adult females, on flower nectar and sap for sustenance. The females mainly use their stinger to subdue cicadas, which they then transport into their underground larders.

They tend to take up residence in high-traffic areas in a yard, probably because of the ease of burrowing along sidewalk and deck edges, as well as in planters and window boxes. But they're mostly just a nuisance. Control is usually a matter of covering holes with sod or rocks and eliminating attractive burrowing areas.

Other hunter wasps more closely fit the general description of the Sphecidae group as the "thread-waisted" wasps. These include the artistically inclined species like the mud dauber, which builds nests of mud on walls and window corners for larvae condos, and the potter wasp, which makes little mud pots with fluted edges for its young.

Like the cicada killer, they hunt other insects to feed to their young, but the adults mostly feed on nectars.

Parasitic Wasps

Parasitic wasps lay their eggs on other living things, like caterpillars or grubs, or insect eggs where, once hatched, the young devour their hosts. Others, like gall wasps, actually produce chemicals that instruct plants to grow special homes for their larvae that provide both shelter and food.

Among the parasitic wasps, the ichneumons, sometimes called ichneumon flies, are the most abundant Hymenoptera species in North America.[22] They are beneficial insects and while their lifestyles are the stuff of nightmares, they're solitary wasps that are generally harmless to people. The same can't be said of their insect prey.

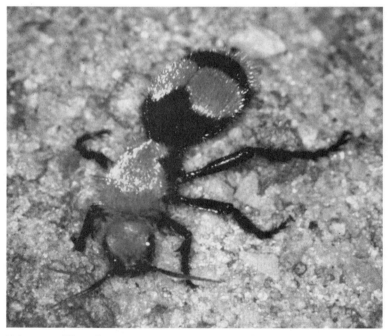

Velvet ant. (Photo by Jerry A. Payne, USDA Agricultural Research Service, Bugwood.org. This work is licensed under a Creative Commons Attribution 3.0 License.)

Braconids are similar to ichneumon wasps but smaller, with contained ovipositors. The minute parasitic wasps, which are among the smallest insects in Florida, are able to complete their entire lifecycle within the tiny egg of hosts like stink bugs and water striders.

A particularly spectacular member of the parasitic wasp group is an insect that looks often nothing like a wasp—the velvet ant, also known as a "cow killer," although it does nothing so drastic as that. The velvet ant is large, nearly an inch in length, and appears "furry" with striking orange and black coloring. Females are wingless, thus the resemblance to ants. They're often seen scurrying along leaf litter, trying to evade flying males or hunting for the burrows of ground-dwelling bees and wasps, upon whose mature larvae they lay their eggs, in classic parasitic wasp fashion.

Although a solitary insect, velvet ants can sting painfully if handled. It's their only defense against lizards, birds, and other predators. They also defend themselves using repellent chemicals, warning noises, and by even playing dead.[23]

The Vespids

The Vespidae family can be a temperamental one. While there are solitary members of this family, it's the large social members that are of interest, importance, and sometimes danger here. The Vespids are typically divided into two groups: the *polistine* or paper wasps, and the *vespine* wasps like yellowjackets and hornets.

Paper Wasps (genus *Polistes*)

There are nine known species of paper wasps in Florida, familiarly known as *polistes*. Their nests are common around the eaves of homes, hanging suspended by a tiny point like little chambered paper ornaments. Only rarely featuring more than 100 cells, nests are protected by fierce guards of anywhere from one or two insects to dozens. While they can exhibit threatening behavior when disturbed, polistes are not especially aggressive, and it's often possible (although unadvisable) to get within a few inches of a nest without incurring wrath.

Only the females sting, although it's hard to tell who's who when they're droning nearby. According to bug expert Arthur Deyrup,

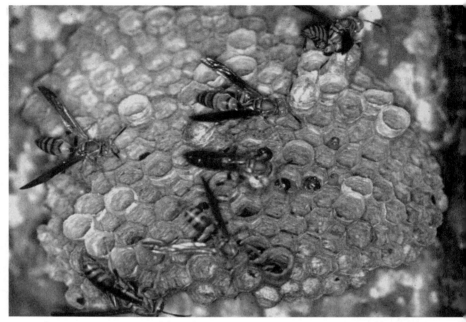

Common paper wasps. (Photo by Jerry A. Payne, USDA Agricultural Research Service.)

male paper wasps will swarm by the dozens around tall trees and man-made structures during the late fall mating season. They seem particularly drawn to a Kennedy Space Center scaffold at Cape Canaveral, where they appear by the hundreds. However, all the high-flying wasps are males and don't sting.

Stings from the females can be painful, but reactions are usually localized. Generalized systemic reactions, while rare, can occur from a paper wasp sting, but since the wasps generally build their nests fairly high, encounters can usually be avoided.

Yellowjackets and Hornets (*Vespula sp.*)

There are actually only three species of vespids in Florida: the eastern yellowjacket (*V. maculifrons*), the southern yellowjacket (*V. squamosal*), and the baldfaced hornet (*Dolichovespula maculate*), which is just another kind of yellowjacket.[24]

All three are highly social insects and aggressive when disturbed.

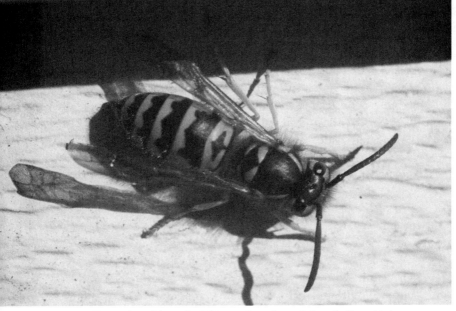

Eastern yellowjacket. (Photo by Whitney Cranshaw, Colorado State University, Bugwood.org. This work is licensed under a Creative Commons Attribution 3.0 License.)

They can be distinguished from one another by variations in color patterns or, in the case of the baldfaced hornet, lack of color. With respect to the similarities of the first two, this begs the usual question regarding things like identifying venomous snakes by the shape of their pupils, namely, "Who hangs around long enough to look that closely?" Most of the time, the names *yellowjacket* and *hornet* are used interchangeably, and the insects are best avoided, whatever the details of their appearance.

Vespids construct elaborate honeycombed nests in trees, on the ground, or underground. Like the polistes, all the vespid nests are made of a papery substance produced by the wasps that is essentially reconstituted wood pulp.[25] In the case of the baldfaced hornet, the nest can be a foot or more in diameter, and while yellowjacket nests traditionally haven't been much larger than a basketball, reports in recent years suggests a troubling change in habits.

One of the largest nests ever discovered was found in Sumter County, Georgia, in 2006. It contained an estimated 100,000 yellowjackets that had nested inside, around, and under the cab of an abandoned truck.[26] In Florida, the largest nest found to date was discovered in Eatonville, also in 2006. It completely encircled a palm tree and contained an estimated 4,000 yellowjackets.[27] Changing weather patterns, including mild winters and drought, are thought to be contributing to these supersized vespid nests.

Housing aside, yellowjackets and hornets ply a similar trade: preying on small insects, which they mash to a pulp with their mandibles and then feed to their larvae. Despite their formidable sting, yellowjackets and hornets do not use their stingers to paralyze prey, but solely as a defensive device. And unlike bees, they can sting repeatedly, which makes mass envenomation from a swarm of angry yellowjackets or hornets a real threat.

While nests usually last only a season or two in colder climates, where the colony dies off during cold weather, in Florida's balmy clime colonies can last two years or more and may possibly signal another adaptation to continuing climate change.

Treating Wasp Stings

As with bees, get away from stinging wasps quickly and calmly, without swatting, and then proceed with treatment for stings. For localized reactions, like pain and swelling at the site of the sting, there are several home remedies that can help.

- Apply an ammonia-based sting treatment. This only works within 15 minutes of a sting by quickly breaking down the protein in the venom.
- Apply ice to area of injury.
- Use an over-the-counter oral antihistamine to reduce reactions.
- Apply hydrocortisone cream to the site of the sting.

For generalized systemic reactions that may include difficulty breathing, swelling of the mouth or throat, body rash, or lightheadedness, head to an emergency room. Clinical treatments will vary with severity of the reaction and can include the following remedies:

- Oral prescription antihistamines
- Injected chlorpheniramine (an antihistamine)
- Intramuscular chlorpheniramine and hydrocortisone
- Inhaled asthma treatments

Immunotherapy for protection against future wasp stings is a consideration if a serious reaction occurs.

As with bees, though, the best treatment is avoidance.

Wasp Habitat

In the natural world, yellowjackets and hornets usually nest underground or at ground level in stumps and logs. With the advent of expanding nest sizes and more varied locations, however, it's clear that wasps are adaptable and will utilize any favorable environment for their nest.

Wasp Control

The best defense for wasps is a good offense. Wasps aren't as frequent flower garden cruisers as bees, and when they do appear, they're likely to be pinching off pesky caterpillars. So gardening won't pose quite the hazard with respect to wasps as it does with bees. Other yard work, however, should be performed cautiously, especially in the summer.

As with bees, it's a good idea to carefully examine work areas before using noisy power equipment in a yard or along tree lines. The vibrations from machines stir up and provoke wasps. Also, regularly inspect the home, especially in the spring and summer, for paper wasp nests along the eaves and for signs of ground nests near highly trafficked areas.

Removing or treating nests is best done at night, preferably with appropriate protective clothing. Nest entrances marked during the day can be dusted with insecticides like Sevin or Ficam and sealed with a shovelful of moist dirt.[28] If there's any doubt at all about the ability to treat a nest, consult professionals. Standing under a nest while trying to remove it goes beyond silly television stunts; it's dangerous, as is accidentally stepping on a nest while trying to remove it, even at night.

Outdoor Safety

Many of the precautions for avoiding bees while outside apply with respect to wasps and hornets.

- Avoid working in flower gardens when hornets and wasps are foraging for nectar.
- Wear shoes when outside, especially in the spring and summer.
- Avoid scented perfumes or lotions.
- Avoid dark clothing, especially blue, which seems to attract wasps and hornets.
- Don't threaten hives by approaching closely or by making loud noises or vibrations.
- Wear appropriate clothing when hiking, including boots or other closed-toed, sturdy footwear, and a hat with neck covering to avoid stings.
- Don't move rapidly or swat at a wasp or yellowjacket; always move slowly and deliberately.
- Keep sweet beverages, foods, and fruits covered when outdoors, and examine drinks or foods before consuming.
- Always have an exit plan!

In Summary

- The insect order Hymenoptera consists of bees, wasps, and ants and includes the majority of stinging and biting insects that produce allergies.
- Reaction to bites and stings takes two forms: Localized reaction includes pain and swelling at the site of injury; generalized systemic response involves allergic reactions, which can vary in severity from hives to anaphylaxis.
- Sting potential is greatest among social bees and wasps. Solitary insects rarely sting unless provoked.
- Of the bees, European and Africanized honeybees are responsible for most stings. Of the two, the Africanized honeybee, also known as the "killer" bee, is the more aggressive.
- Bees leave their stinger in the victim, where it continues to

pump venom until emptied or removed. The method of removal is less important than promptness.

- Of the wasps, paper wasps, yellowjackets, and hornets are the most aggressive and the most likely to sting when their nests are disturbed.
- Avoiding bees and wasps—the principal way to prevent stings—is best accomplished by being aware of one's environment, using caution when operating noisy, vibrating yard equipment, and performing routine walks around house and yard to remove and treat nests as they appear.
- Other precautions include avoiding the use of perfumes and fragrances, wearing light-colored and activity-appropriate clothing, wearing closed-toed shoes, and covering up sweetened foods when dining outdoors.
- Don't swat at bees and wasps; this tends to excite them and may provoke rather than discourage stings.
- Treat stings with an ammonia-based sting neutralizer, clean with soap and water, and apply ice or cold compresses. An antihistamine will reduce reactions further.
- Signs of a severe allergic reaction can include any of the following: difficulty breathing, profuse swelling, extensive hives, nausea, abdominal pain, and/or drop in blood pressure and unconsciousness. At the first sign of any of these reactions, seek immediate medical treatment.

Hymenoptera, Part II

The Ants

> Karl Marx was right, socialism works,
> it is just that he had the wrong species.
>
> Edward O. Wilson, *The Ants*

Most of the 221 known ant species in Florida are harmless to people. Of the half dozen or so that sting or bite (or both), the red imported fire ant (RIFA) or *Solenopsis invicta*, is responsible for more allergy problems than any ant, or any other member of the Hymenoptera family. Over 40 percent of Hymenoptera venom hypersensitivity cases in the southeastern United States are attributable to fire ant stings.[1] And the unavoidable fact is that almost everyone in Florida is eventually stung by fire ants.

The Red Imported Fire Ant (RIFA)—Allergy Potential: Moderate to High

Of Florida's more than 200 ant species, 52 are exotics, comprising the largest number of exotic ant species anywhere in the United States. Among them, RIFA may be the most problematic. A native South American ant that made its way to the United States via Mobile, Alabama, in the 1930s, today it infests more than 300 million acres across the southeastern and southwestern United States, and continues to spread.[2]

The toll the species takes on wildlife, agriculture, and human society in general in Florida is significant, costing homeowners and businesses $25 to $40 million annually in chemical fire ant pesticides alone. That doesn't even take into consideration the costs for doctor visits, antihistamines, and immunological treatments. In South America, RIFA are kept in check by other competitive ant species, natural predators, and native pathogens. The United States apparently lacks any of these natural controls, and so RIFA spread at a population rate of five times more ants per acre here than in their native habitat in South America.[3]

RIFA are almost indistinguishable from other fire ant species, including our native fire ant, a less aggressive and beneficial insect that could help keep RIFA in check if it isn't accidentally eradicated in the full frontal assault on its imported cousin. RIFA have shiny reddish-orange heads and black abdomens, and like many fire ant species, they vary widely in length, ranging from a tenth of an inch to nearly half an inch in length depending on their job in the colony.

Minutely distinguishing features can be identified by ant specialists with magnifying glasses, but for our purposes, their most identifying characteristic is the clearly visible stingers on the tips of their abdomens, which only workers possess, and their telltale mounds. Adding insult to injury, fire ants actually both bite and sting, first attaching to the skin with their mandibles and then administering their venomous sting.

Fire ant venom is distinct from the venom of wasps, bees, and hornets, although some cross-reactivity with other fire ants as well as with other Hymenoptera venom has been reported. RIFA venom has a low protein content and a high concentration (up to 95 percent) of water-insoluble alkaloids, the component responsible for the pain and the nasty little pustule that forms a few hours to a day after the sting.[4]

The 5 percent aqueous portion of the venom contains major allergenic proteins that can cause serious systemic reactions in about 2 percent of the victims who have sought help. Reactions can include flushing, urticaria (hives), and angiodema (swelling of the mouth and lips).[5]

Scratching at the itchy pustules can cause them to break and become infected, causing further problems. And allergies to RIFA can develop fairly quickly.

Wynn Wargo, of Clearwater, experienced the suddenness of a RIFA allergy with her 5-year-old daughter, Joy. Dared by another child to sit on a RIFA mound, Joy was roundly stung, although by fewer ants than in previous encounters, her mother recalls. Concerned by the reaction her daughter seemed to be having, Wargo took her to the nearest emergency room.

"Before we drove 100 feet," Wargo said, "she was coughing and choking in the back seat. I was by myself, so it was hard to comfort her and drive at the same time."

As Joy's condition deteriorated, Wargo stopped at a drugstore to buy some Benadryl for her before continuing on to the hospital. But spotting a sheriff's deputy nearby, Wargo alerted him and he called 911.

"Her blood pressure was dropping, but they tried to assure me that everything would be okay. There was an intense phone consult with the local emergency department. The techs were ordered to give her a dose of a powerful antihistamine. They presented her with a stuffed spider and delivered us to the emergency department door. Her condition was monitored for several hours after her blood pressure stabilized."

The next day, the family pediatrician informed Wargo that her daughter had suffered a life-threatening reaction to fire ant bites and referred them to a pediatric allergist.

"Our daughter will need to carry an Epi-Pen for the rest of her life," said Wargo.

RIFA are adaptable, omnivorous, voracious, easily provoked, and extremely aggressive. They will sting individually or en mass, pouring out of a disturbed mound seeking high ground along leaf blades and legs to sting everything and anything within reach.

Although it's quite possible to find oneself standing in a sea of RIFA with no mound in sight, in most cases the mound is spotted first. A visible mound is at least six months old and contains several thousand workers. The queen produces eggs at the prodigious rate of about 1,500 per day. RIFA colonies may contain multiple queens, called polygyne colonies, and produce up to 1,000 mounds per acre sheltering an astonishing 40 million ants.[6]

Mounds can grow to two feet in diameter and up to eight inches in height. In clay soils, nests have been known to reach three feet in height and have galleries extending up to six feet below ground. A mature mound can contain nearly a quarter of a million ants.[7] RIFA mounds are coned like those of most ants, but lack a central opening at the top. Instead, RIFA have multiple entrances to their main mound, identifiable by irregularly scattered soil nearby.

While they prefer dry open areas, RIFA will also nest under concrete slabs, in lawns, along sidewalk edges, in electrical boxes and inside water pumps. They'll eat everything from the early, tender growth of crops like citrus, beans, corn, cabbage, cucumber, and

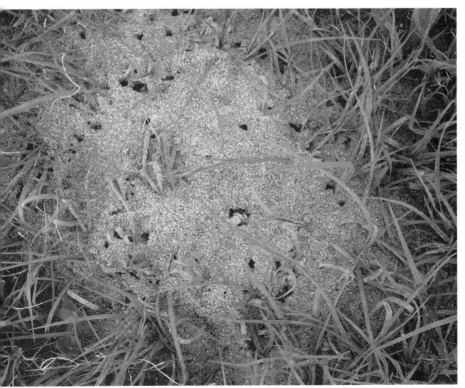

Red imported fire ant mound. (Photo by Theresa Willingham.)

potatoes to endangered gopher tortoises and ground nesting birds, seriously impacting populations of both.

If the red imported fire ant seems completely irredeemable, that may be the case. While the other insects examined so far have some place in nature, even renowned Florida entomologist Mark Deyrup is unable to find much of a silver lining in the red imported fire ant cloud. "Biologists see no redeeming features of fire ants in Florida habitats. . . . In Florida, fire ants reduce the populations of many native insects, and attack helpless vertebrates, such as ground nesting birds just hatching from the egg. In lawns, gardens, and fields, fire ants are a nuisance because of their aggressiveness."[8]

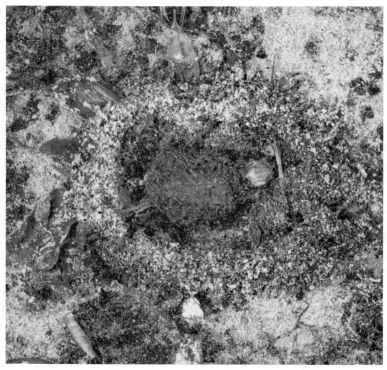

Newly hatched turtle killed by red imported fire ants. (Photo by Theresa Willingham.)

Other Stinging or Biting Ants—Allergy Potential: Mild to Moderate, Depending on Species

While RIFA is clearly the most problematic ant in the state, it is not the only biting and stinging ant in Florida, nor the only one known to cause allergies. At least six subfamilies of ants are capable of causing adverse or allergic reactions in people.[9]

Besides RIFA, most people will have run-ins with only four or five other principal biting ant species in Florida, namely, the little fire ant, native tropical fire ant, Florida harvester ant, Mexican, or elongate, twig ant, and the carpenter ant.

Little Fire Ant (*Wasmannia auropunctata*)

The little fire ant is another import, hailing from northern and central South America and the West Indies. Tiny at about an eighth of an inch and golden in color, its preferred nesting habit is the soil under leaf debris, old logs, around the base of trees, and in clumps of grass—the shared habitat of the Florida gardener.[10] It possesses a disproportionately painful sting for its size, with the sensation of the sting building slowly and lasting for up to fifteen minutes.[11]

The little fire ant is most common in South and Central Florida, where it can infest citrus groves and wreak havoc on grove workers because of its habit of stinging when trapped under clothing, as well as when caught in droplets of sweat on the skin. In homes, the little fire ant will infest items of clothing, beds, furniture, or oily foods like peanut butter.

Tropical Fire Ant (*Solenopsis geminate*)

Not that the little and red imported fire ants leave much room for it, but Florida has a native version, the tropical fire ant. A reddish brown ant one-third of an inch long, it builds irregular crater-shaped mounds in disturbed, sunny areas. Like the other fire ants, workers of this species can and do sting when disturbed, and rather painfully, but they're less aggressive than RIFA.

Also like many other ants, the native makes its living tending honeydew-producing insects, primarily mealy bugs. It's alternately considered an important species, for its competitiveness with the more virulent red imported fire ant, and a nuisance because, like RIFA, it has a nasty sting and its honeydew habit contributes to the propagation of crop pests.[12]

Twig Ant (*Seudomyrmex gracilis*)

Another import, the twig ant, also known as the elongate twig ant, is an arboreal Mexican species somewhat resembling a wingless wasp. About half an inch long and orange and black in color, the twig ant feeds on live insects and fungus spores and tends aphids for honeydew which, in turn, draws gardeners trying to eliminate the aphids, bringing human necks and frantic ants into unfortunate contact.[13]

While their sting is painful, twig ants aren't aggressive. They often fall onto gardeners and outdoors people unnoticed. It's only when a hapless human suddenly feels something crawling along his or her neck and starts swatting that the twig ant is provoked into self-defensive stinging, earning it the nickname "neck-biter ant."[14] The sting hurts and usually leaves a significant welt, but no allergies appear to be associated with twig ant stings.

Florida Harvester Ant (*Pogonomyrmex badius*)

The Florida harvester ant is a seed collector with a yen for ant mound feng shui. It also has a disproportionately wicked sting, hailing from a family of ants with a reputation for having the most potent venom of any insect, comparable to cobra venom in strength.[15] Harvester ants are fairly common, although *P. badius* is the only harvester ant east of the Mississippi, and despite its potent sting, it is a decidedly passive ant and less "badius" than its name would suggest.

The Florida harvester ant is an interesting species with unique home improvement habits. It prefers open sandy areas for its nest, usually in open woodlands or light grassy areas. Mounds are modest, with single or multiple entrances in the center, but well decorated, as the harvester ant likes to cover its nest with small pebbles, twigs, and bits of charcoal.[16]

Although the ant almost has to be forced to sting, the few reports of stings are sobering.[17]

A 1938 description of an encounter with harvester ants reads,

"Several ants stung me on the wrist, and after a few minutes an intense fiery pain began in this area which was about two inches in diameter. It turned deep red in color and immediately a watery, sticky secretion came out of the skin. This area became hot and feverish and the excruciating pain lasted all day and up into the night."[18]

One death, of a child in Oklahoma in the 1990s, has been attributed to the red harvester ant, *P. barbatus*.[19]

Yet despite the volatile potential of this insect, the harvester ant is not considered a species of concern with respect to allergies. Nests are rarely encountered in suburban Florida, and the ants simply aren't aggressive in accidental encounters.

Florida Carpenter Ant (*Camponotus abdominalis floridanus*)

The carpenter ant is another species more daunting in appearance than it is in reality. These are the largest ants in Florida, measuring nearly half an inch in length. With a yellow and red thorax, shiny black abdomen, and determined scurry, carpenter ants certainly look lethal.

They make their nests in mulch, logs, and wall areas of homes, but despite their name, they do not damage wood like the Panhandle's black carpenter ant or western U.S. carpenter ants. Instead, carpenter ants capitalize on woods already softened or damaged by wood rot or termites, providing evidence of existing damage rather than being the cause of it. Nevertheless, 20 percent of homeowner complaints about ants in the greater metropolitan areas of Florida concern carpenter ants.[20]

Carpenter ants don't sting, but they do bite with their sturdy mandibles, and while the bite may be painful, it's not known to cause allergic reactions.

Treating Ant Bites and Stings

Localized reactions to ant bites and stings are treated like those of most other Hymenoptera encounters.

- Within 15 minutes of a sting, if possible, apply an ammonia-based sting treatment, which helps break down the protein in fire ant venom.

- Wash the area with soap and water.
- Apply cool compresses.
- Take over-the-counter oral antihistamines or apply cortico-steroid creams for itching and swelling.[21]

For multiple stings or if a more generalized reaction occurs, visit a doctor or emergency room. If anaphylaxis threatens, injectable epinephrine will be ordered and prescribed to keep on hand against future encounters.

If serious reactions to red ant stings are a problem, an allergist or immunologist should be consulted for more extensive skin or in vitro testing for fire ant hypersensitivity. Such hypersensitivity is usually indicated by any one of the following experiences:

- Emergency treatment for fire ant stings
- An experience of anaphylaxis, with a fire ant sting as a possible cause
- A coexisting condition that may complicate treatment of anaphylaxis (e.g., using beta-blockers, having hypertension or cardiac arrhythmias)

Treatments in the case of severe allergy to ant stings can include the prescription of the injectable epinephrine and possibly venom immunotherapy, including Rush (accelerated) Immunotherapy (RIT).[22] Being familiar with ant habitats and creating less welcoming environments for them, though, can go a long way toward avoiding problems in the first place.

Ant Habitats

Ants can live just about anywhere, as any frustrated homeowner can confirm who finds them thriving in a laundry hamper, in a pet food dish, or in a medicine cabinet enjoying the cough syrup. With the exception of the little fire ant, though, most of the biting and stinging ants have pretty specific outdoor habitats and habits that education can help you avoid.

Ants typically establish new colonies in two main ways:

1. Annual or semiannual swarms of winged reproductive ants
2. Budding, where one or more queens leaves the nest with a contingent of workers

Common household ants, like the Pharaoh and ghost ants, and some fire ants spread via budding. Most ant species spread via swarming flight.

Ants are essentially omnivorous, feasting on everything from other insects to seeds, oils, sugar, and honeydew. Food is located by randomly searching scout ants. When a scout encounters food, it will take a piece or the whole thing back to the nest, leaving a scent trail there and back to the food source.[23] Bites and stings occur when we cross paths, however inadvertently, with foraging or nesting ants.

As with most Hymenoptera, being aware of nests is a critical part of avoiding accidental encounters. RIFA live in areas of disturbed land, in colonies of large dome-shaped mounds with multiple entrances, sometimes barely visible as nearby areas of scattered sand or soil, and no central opening. Most of their foraging actually occurs underground.

Unfortunately, they tend to nest in areas people have disturbed for their own purposes, like gardens, yards, parks, and playgrounds. They're also common in agricultural fields (where gopher mounds, which are much larger and usually far more numerous, are often confused for RIFA nests). Suburban encounters are the most problematic, though, and occur when RIFA nest under patio slabs, along sidewalks and driveways, and inside electrical equipment.[24]

Little fire ants tend to forage along sidewalks and building foundations. They make their way into homes and buildings via landscape timbers and stones, where they continue their treks along baseboards and under the edges of carpets.

Carpenter ants are mostly outdoor or structural pests and will usually enter homes only for water and sometimes food, depending on developmental needs, which vary by season: protein during brood development in the spring and summer, and carbohydrates during late summer and fall.[25]

At-Risk Populations

There are several risk factors that can lead to serious situations between people and stinging ants, especially RIFA. Of course, accidental encounters near nests in yards or playgrounds are common. But immobility is another, seemingly incongruous risk factor that leads to serious ant sting problems in Florida, especially among the elderly.

Nursing home infestations of RIFA are common, especially as drought conditions force ants indoors in search of water or flood conditions force them in for dry ground. Several wrongful death suits have been filed in recent years as a result of RIFA attacks in nursing homes.

Most notable is the nearly $2 million wrongful death settlement in 2001 to the family of a 73-year-old retired postal worker who died of shock after being stung repeatedly by red fire ants. The ants swarmed his hospital bed in an Atlantic Shores nursing home where he was recovering from surgery. Records showed that the nursing home had battled fire ant infestations for years.[26]

But deaths and severe reactions associated with nursing homes and limited-mobility victims such as infants, the inebriated, or those who've fallen asleep near mounds are more often due to mass envenomation than allergies. Those with compromised immune systems or with poor circulation or neurosensation (such as diabetes mellitus sufferers) are also at risk. People at greatest risk for allergic responses are typically those who've had previous sensitization exposure.

Ant Control

Preventing indoor ant infestations and controlling immediate outdoor populations are the best ways to remain safe from injury or allergy problems with respect to ants around homes, buildings, and other commonly used outdoor areas. Recommended indoor prevention measures include the following:

- Keep floors and counters free of food particles and liquids.
- Remove or regularly treat indoor plants that can harbor ants, aphids, whiteflies, or other honeydew-producing insects.
- Repair or control any indoor condensation or leaks.[27]

To protect infants, the elderly, or the infirm from fire ant injury at home or in managed-care facilities, it's important to take simple precautions:

- Keep linens off the floor and beds away from walls.
- Discourage eating in bed, and check mattresses regularly for food particles.
- Keep all food in closed, airtight containers.
- Keep medicines and fluids well sealed.
- Vacuum regularly.

Outdoors, a couple of interesting biological controls exist: armadillos and phorid flies. Armadillos act essentially as Florida anteaters, digging into fire ant mounds with apparent impunity to chow down on the developing ant broods that inhabit the top portions of the mounds. Unfortunately, they tend to eat fire ants as a last resort and not in sufficient numbers to reduce populations.[28]

The phorid fly seems the most promising candidate so far. In May 2009, after decades of study, Texas researchers released a new and improved species of phorid fly to combat RIFA there, inspiring the lurid headline, "Ants Become Headless Zombies."[29] The phorid fly under study in Texas and in Florida is a tiny parasitic insect that lays its eggs on a specific host, in this case, only red imported fire ants.

When an egg hatches, the larval maggot proceeds to feast inside its host's head until it literally decapitates the ant. The zombie reference is apropos, as the ant wanders aimlessly for up to two weeks before its head falls off and a new phorid fly emerges to find more ants upon which to lay eggs. The RIFA phorid fly has a taste only for RIFA and does not harm any native ants, including the tropical fire ant. The phorid fly species tested in 2009 is an improvement over past introductions because the fly attacks ants away from their mound, as opposed to only being attracted to the mound itself.

Unfortunately, armadillos aren't particularly reliable, and it will take another few decades to know exactly how effective phorid fly controls are. Instead, a more reliable solution is to take steps to clear the immediate 25 to 50 feet around the outside of a building:

- Maintain 18 to 20 inches of clear air space between the building and the mature height and width of ornamental plants.

- Aim sprinkler heads away from buildings as much as possible to minimize moisture on walls.
- Grade yards to slope away from buildings to prevent pooling of water along foundations.
- Ensure downspouts drain away from building foundations.
- Treat yards regularly for ants—new once-a-year products are proving fairly successful (for now) at reducing RIFA mounds in yards.[30]

Beyond prevention, there are two main ways to treat for ants: baits and chemical controls.[31] Baits work by taking advantage of most ants'

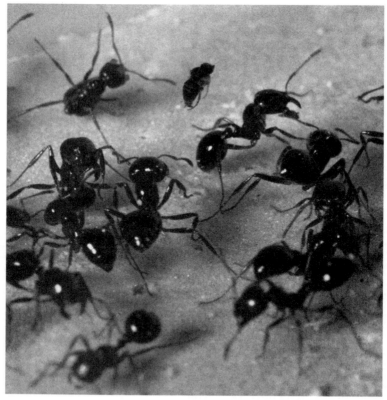

Phorid fly attacking red imported fire ants. (Photo by Scott Bauer, USDA Agricultural Research Service.)

devotion to their queens, to whom they bring predigested food that they feed her directly. Most baits consist of a slow-acting insecticide (so it doesn't kill the workers carrying the bait back to the queen) and some type of vegetable oil base. There are a wide variety of baits available, but a good home brew is one teaspoon of boric acid heated and dissolved in 2 ½ ounces of corn syrup or honey and diluted with an equal amount of water. The bait can then be applied with an eye dropper along known trails or feeding areas. Be sure to keep it out of reach of children.

Chemical controls vary widely, available as liquids, powders, dusts, and granules that can be applied directly to observed mounds. They're more effective for species like carpenter ants. Chemical pesticides must be used carefully to avoid eradicating beneficial insects or poisoning pets and people. Used properly, however, they can create an effective barrier between home and yard.

Outdoor Protection

Outdoor safety is a matter of being observant and, evidently, of wearing socks. In one study, researchers fitted commercially available infant socks over plastic doll feet and stretched socks and cotton tights over their fingers to test the ability of ants to sting through fabric.

The results showed that "socks of any type reduced the number of fire ants that reached the skin and delayed the time required for ants to reach the skin above the sock level. Fire ants were unable to sting through all socks tested." Researchers also observed that RIFA were undeterred by chemical skin repellents.

Consequently, the researchers concluded, "Socks provide some degree of protection from fire ant stings; therefore, children living in fire ant-infested areas should wear them."[32]

And probably hikers and other outdoors people as well, although plenty of sock-wearing Floridians will point out that socks may also slow cognizance of standing on an ant pile, delaying the inevitable bites rather than significantly thwarting them.

That said, wearing socks and closed-toed shoes, as opposed to the stylish Florida look of socks with sandals, may significantly protect against ant bites and is recommended for all hikers, fishermen, and gardeners. Here is some more advice:

- Look before you sit or sleep. Avoid sitting on rotten logs or kicking apart stumps. Lots of insects, including ants, make their homes in decomposing stumps and logs. Check areas thoroughly before settling in for picnics or camping.
- Wear gloves when working in gardens or outdoor areas, or near electrical boxes, where ants might be present.
- Dust gloves, lower extremities, tool areas, bird nesting boxes, and other possibly attractive ant areas with talcum powder (ineffective in high humidity).
- Keep food well sealed, indoors and out.
- Keep antihistamines and sting treatments available, regardless of known allergies or lack of them, for use in the event of multiple stings.
- Don't swat ants. Brush and sweep them off if they sting you, and move quickly away from the area.[33]

In Summary

- Of the 221 known ant species in Florida, only six sting and/or bite: the red imported fire ant (RIFA), the little fire ant, the tropical fire ant, the Mexican twig ant, the Florida harvester ant, and, occasionally, the carpenter ant.
- Of the stinging ants, RIFA causes the most allergy problems. Among not only the ants but among all other Hymenoptera, RIFA is responsible for more than 40 percent of Hymenoptera venom hypersensitivity cases in the southeastern U.S.
- RIFA prefer nesting in dry open areas but will also nest under concrete slabs, in lawns, along sidewalk edges, in electrical boxes and water pumps. They will eat everything from tender young crops to the young of ground-nesting birds.
- As with bees and wasps, response to ant bites takes two forms: localized reactions that include pain and swelling at

the injury site or generalized systemic response in the form of allergic reactions.

- Those at greatest risk for injury by RIFA include people with limited mobility, people with compromised immune systems, people with poor circulation or neurosensation, and people who have had previous sensitization exposure.
- Prevention of ant bites is the best control and includes measures like keeping home surfaces free of food particles and moisture, removing indoor plants that may harbor aphids or other honeydew-producing insects that ants "farm," sealing leaks, and storing foods and fluids, including medicines, in airtight containers.
- Outdoor controls include maintaining 18 to 20 inches of clear space around buildings and plants, aiming sprinklers away from buildings, ensuring water doesn't pool near foundations, and treating regularly for ants with baits or chemical controls.
- Outdoor safety includes wearing shoes, not sitting on or kicking apart old logs or stumps, and wearing gloves and socks when working outdoors or hiking.
- Treat stings with an ammonia-based sting neutralizer, cleanse with soap and water, and apply ice or cold compresses. An antihistamine will reduce reactions further.
- Signs of severe allergic reaction can include any of the following: difficulty breathing, profuse swelling, extensive hives, nausea, abdominal pain, and/or drop in blood pressure and unconsciousness. At the first sign of any of these reactions, seek immediate medical treatment.

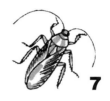

La Cucaracha

Cockroach Allergy Potential—Surprisingly High

> Both the cockroach and the bird would get along very well
> without us, although the cockroach would miss us most.
>
> Joseph Wood Krutch

Few creatures evoke such fear and loathing as the cockroach. And in the continuing irony of life in Florida, few creatures are so perfectly adapted to living here.

Of the order Blattaria (Latin for "insect that shuns the light") and relatively unchanged over the last 300 million years, the cockroach is the ultimate survivor. Able to withstand extremes in temperature, diet, and environment, it is aided in its survival by an uneasy alliance with humans. Constantly striving to eradicate it, we are also unwitting but often enabling partners in its success.

Although most people will see only 3 or 4 common species of cockroaches in and around their homes, typically the American, Australian, and German cockroaches, nearly 40 cockroach species live in Florida. Most prefer the outdoors, living in damp, moldering environments among rotten logs, grasses, and leaf litter.

The cockroach "yuck" factor is admittedly high among both residents and visitors, causing not only consternation and stress among the Blattodephobic and casual roach hater alike but also real health threats from contamination of food with cockroach excrement and the spread of pathogenic disease.

But it is the cockroach's allergy potential that we're looking at here, which turns out to be significant. It's estimated that more than 26 percent of Americans exhibit allergic sensitivity to the German cockroach, the most common indoor variety.[1]

Of greater significance is how that allergy seems to manifest itself in growing numbers of asthma cases. Asthma has been on the increase since 1980, coinciding, notes the Environmental Protection Agency, with Americans' growing tendency to stay indoors, in far more tightly insulated homes that not only provide climate control but also trap allergens. Studies on indoor allergens have established exposure to cockroaches and their allergens as a significant risk factor for asthma, especially in children, where up to 80 percent of those with asthma may have IgE antibodies to cockroach allergens.[2]

The National Cooperative Inner-City Asthma Study (NCICAS), a landmark National Institute of Allergy and Infectious Diseases (NI-AID) study begun in 1996, found that children were more allergic to cockroaches (37 percent) than to dust mites (35 percent) or cats (23 percent).[3] The problem was greater in northeastern cities than in southern locales, where dust mites are a bigger problem. But in all cases, failure to control cockroaches in homes can exacerbate or trigger asthma in children and, less commonly, in adults.

How Cockroaches Cause Allergies

Okay, sit down and try not to get queasy. Here's the scoop from the Asthma and Allergy Foundation of America (AAFA). Cockroach allergens are carried in the saliva, fecal waste, body secretions, cast skins, and brittle carcasses of cockroaches. They can trigger allergic responses in hypersensitive individuals that range from skin rashes from actual contact with the insects to respiratory problems like asthma due to inhalation of minute particles of cockroach skin, fecal, or other material.[4]

The allergens of the two most commonly found indoor cockroaches, the German (*B. germanica*) and the American cockroach

(*P. americana*), have been identified through sequencing and cloning and, like most cockroach allergens, found to be species-specific.[5] The main cockroach allergens, known chemically as "Bla g 1" and "Bla g 2," act directly on the respiratory and bronchial airway systems where they cause inflammation and constriction.[6]

Cockroach allergy can result after an initial exposure to the insect's allergenic components through inhalation, ingestion, or actual contact. Sensitive individuals react to roach allergens at 2 to 8 units (80 to 160 nanograms) per gram (U/g) of dust. In a nationally representative sample, researchers found that 11 percent of U.S. living rooms and 13 percent of U.S. kitchens exceed 2 U/g of cockroach allergens. Detectable concentrations of allergens (>0.4 U/g) were found in over 27 percent of homes.[7]

Although a lot of people show sensitization to cockroach allergens, not everyone will develop an allergy to them. Most susceptible are those with chronic severe bronchial asthma, chronic rhinitis, sinus infections, and ear infections. Symptoms can include itchy skin and irritated scratchy throat, nose, or eyes.[8]

Sometimes the only sign will be persistent year-round asthma, as opposed to seasonal asthma. The National Heart, Lung, and Blood Institute, which takes these things seriously, urges anyone suffering from chronic asthma or other persistent inflammatory or respiratory symptoms to be tested for cockroach allergy. Diagnosis is made at an allergist's office via a skin test.

An Inevitable Association

Homeowners who are neat and tidy and haven't seen a cockroach in ages can probably rest assured they don't have serious infestations. But for homeowners living in Florida, chances are better than average that there are still cockroaches in even the neatest homes, especially in urban areas.

The AAFA cites studies suggesting that 78–98 percent of urban homes harbor cockroaches ranging in number from 900 to more than 300,000. The creepy rule of thumb is that for every roach seen inside, one can safely assume there are at least 800 others dwelling out of sight somewhere nearby.

Roaches typically come into homes in shopping bags, luggage, or potted plants, through open doors or windows, in furniture, and in any items brought in from outside. They'll also take up residence in an apartment or multifamily housing unit if a neighboring unit is infested.

Florida Cockroaches

Garden-variety cockroaches in Florida consist mainly of the following (listed in order of decreasing size):

- Florida woods roach
- American
- Australian
- Brown
- Smoky brown
- Brown banded
- German
- Asian[9]

The observant reader will notice "palmetto bug" is not on the list. That's because "palmetto bug," usually uttered as an exclamation, is actually a colloquial term for cockroaches often applied with equal fervor and dismay to any large, winged roach spied scurrying across a floor or fluttering haphazardly across a room.

All roaches are pretty much naturalized citizens, hailing from around the world, adapting to the environment of the moment, hitching rides to everywhere else on land and sea throughout the ages. Even their common names belie their international ancestry: the "American" and the "Australian" cockroaches are African in origin, and the "German" cockroach is Asian.[10] What all cockroaches do have in common is adaptability, hardiness, speed, agility, and a remarkably omnivorous appetite.

They also have some really impressive cerci, a pair of stiff hairs on the ends of their abdomens that act as very finely tuned touch sensors. Cerci are most evident on insects like earwigs. But the cockroach cerci are so sensitive to movement—like the undetectable rush of air from your uplifted foot before it comes to bear on a hapless insect—that they stimulate nerve fibers at an astounding speed, causing the roach to whisk away before it even knows why, and thereby making it almost impossible to stomp.

Life of the Cockroach

Cockroaches have three stages of life: egg, nymph, and adult. Cockroach eggs develop in a leathery double-rowed purselike case called an ootheca. Females typically drop or glue the case to some surface as soon as it is formed, except for the German cockroach, which will carry the case protruding from its body until the eggs are ready to hatch.

Newly hatched nymphs are wingless and pale in color, often mistaken for white cockroaches. They molt several times before adulthood. Outdoor cockroaches like the Florida woods roach may take up to a year to develop into an adult, but indoor German and brown banded cockroaches may produce several generations in a year, and given the number of eggs in a German cockroach's ootheca, that's a lot of cockroaches.

Larger species of cockroaches can live up to two years, producing an egg case containing 10–28 eggs about every week or two. The German cockroach ootheca contains 30–40 eggs, double that of other species.[11]

The Florida Woods Roach (*Eurycotis floridana*)

Of the big cockroaches, the Florida woods roach is, in fact, a native, palmetto-dwelling variety and the largest of our local Blattaria, measuring up to two inches long. It has a distinctly prehistoric appearance, from its large armored, troglodyte build to its lumbering gait.

The Florida woods roach is also known as the Florida stinkroach or skunkroach, for its propensity to emit, when startled, an oily odiferous liquid from its underbelly. While the scent is said to "stink," ever since a friend suggested it actually smells like cherries, that's all I've ever smelled in the presence of a woods roach. Others say the scent is like amaretto. Either way, like most outdoors roaches, the Florida woods roach does not survive well indoors and is unlikely to produce any allergies.

The American Cockroach (*P. americana*)

The American cockroach is a significant species in cockroach allergies, second only to the German cockroach in abundance. Also known as a water bug, flying water bug, or palmetto bug, it is the largest of the roaches commonly found indoors, measuring up to an inch and a half in length. American cockroaches are reddish brown with a pale brown or yellow band around the edge of the pronotum (front top surface of the thorax). Males' wings extend beyond their abdomens, making them somewhat longer than the females.

American cockroaches coexist with German cockroaches and live as equally comfortably outdoors as in. They can be found in caves, mines, latrines, cesspools, sewers, treatment plants, and dumps, where they pick up bacteria, viruses, fungi, protozoa, and even helminthic worms, all of which they can transport and transmit.

They're resistant to some insecticides, can live a month without food or water, and are able to eat virtually anything, including paper, hair, soft leather, beer, and especially anything sweet.[12] They're also an anathema for their tendency to leave trails of excrement and regurgitation in their wake. Their resilience makes them a difficult indoor pest to conquer.

Australian Cockroach (*Periplaneta australasiae*)

Australian cockroaches are about the same size as the American cockroach, reddish brown in color with a distinctive coloration on the top of the head: two dark spots in a field of pale yellow or tan. There's also a light yellow band along the front edge of the forewing. Australian cockroaches are common in greenhouses and gardens and can damage plants. They can also make their way indoors, but are not considered a significant allergenic species like the American and German cockroaches.

Smoky Brown Cockroach (*Periplaneta fuliginosa*)

The smoky brown cockroach is about 1¼ inches in length, a fairly solid mahogany brown to black, with few other visible markings or patterns. It's primarily an outdoor species, common among wood piles and tree holes, but can be driven indoors by inclement weather. Indoors, it's often found in attics around the roof line. While its usual diet consists of decaying vegetation, it'll eat anything any other pest cockroach eats indoors.[13]

German Cockroach (*B. germanica*)

German cockroaches are similar in size and appearance to the Asian (although the Asian is rarely found indoors) and brown banded cockroaches, relatively small at about a half inch in length and extraordinarily prolific, producing double the offspring of other cockroach species. They're considered a significant pest roach, residing in dark, warm, close, and humid crevices near food and water sources and, unlike many other species of cockroach, able to breed indoors.

They rarely come out into the open, preferring to travel along enclosed spaces and structures, and seldom in the daytime. Seeing a German cockroach indoors during the day is a good indication that

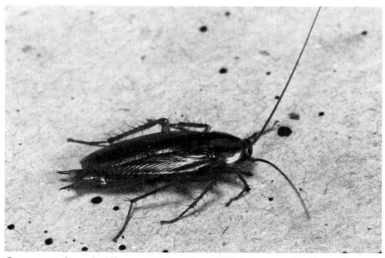

German cockroach. (Clemson University—USDA Cooperative Extension Slide Series, Bugwood.org. This work is licensed under a Creative Commons Attribution 3.0 License.)

large populations of them have taken up residence, as is the sight of completely white nymphs and adults.[14] The German cockroach will dine on everything from grease and soap to glue and toothpaste.

Brown Banded Cockroach (*Supella longipalpa*)

Brown banded cockroaches are dark brown with two pale brown bands on the wings. They like height and warmth and can be found around motors, clocks, televisions, and shower stalls, usually along the upper reaches of walls, on shelves, and around ceiling fixtures. Unlike the German cockroach, they don't require freestanding water and prefer starchy materials, including book bindings and wallpapers. They're active roaches, and both genders of the species fly.

Newcomers

In 2008, entomologists issued warnings about exotic cockroaches making their way into Florida via the herpetology hobby trade, as a result of a new trend in reptile feeding practices.[15] In recent years, hobbyists turned from farming crickets to feed their lizards, to cockroaches, since, as might be expected, roaches are cheap and easy to raise, as well as quiet and less odiferous than crickets.

The major exotic imports by herpetologists are the Turkestan, Madagascar hissing cockroach, lobster roach, and orange spotted roach. None of these are currently established in Florida, although the Turkestan has apparently carved out a comfortable living in Texas, New Mexico, and Arizona, after inadvertent import by U.S. military personnel and equipment returning from the Middle East.

The Madagascar hissing cockroach is an enormous species, measuring up to three inches in length and, as its name suggests, of a more loquacious nature than most cockroaches. It's definitely not something Floridians would like to find in their homes. For the time being, entomologists are counseling awareness, and pest control specialists are on the lookout for unusual species encountered during their normal rounds.

Treating Cockroach Allergy

As with all allergies, treatment for cockroach allergy involves a three-pronged approach, beginning with prevention, which in this case consists of cleanliness and control. Eliminating roach habitat by keeping surfaces, corners, and crevices clean and dry is the best way to reduce, if not eliminate, cockroaches and their commensurate allergenic waste in homes and businesses.

For uncontrolled exposure that might occur in schools, businesses, medical facilities, and other environments where cockroaches may be a contributing factor in asthma and allergy symptoms, the second prong of treatment utilizes antihistamines, decongestants, and anti-inflammatory and bronchodilators to help reduce reactions.

Immunotherapy, the third approach, traditionally has not proven very effective in the alleviation and control of cockroach allergies. However, treatment with cockroach extracts is under study with the hopes of creating better immunotherapy treatments.[16] A trial begun in 2007 and expected to conclude in 2014 is evaluating the safety and efficacy of—if one can stomach the thought—a sublingual cockroach extract as well.[17]

Controlling cockroaches, though, remains the principal way of reducing exposure to related allergens and commensurate symptoms.

Control

Outdoors, cockroaches are kept in check by natural predators, like parasitic wasps that lay eggs on the ootheca, and the swift and enormous huntsman spider, with its five-inch leg span. There are a number of residential controls and practices, however, that homeowners can take.

- Maintain cleanliness by storing food in airtight containers; keep floors, counters, and cabinets free of food particles or other organic materials; and keep trash cans closed and regularly emptied.
- Reduce access to water by sealing leaks, wrapping pipes to reduce condensation, eliminating damp areas including wet,

damaged wood and damp laundry, and removing wet leaves around house foundations.

- Eliminate hiding areas by removing household clutter, including piles of newspapers, magazines, and laundry, and cleaning out sinks, cabinets, and shelves.
- Eliminate cockroach entryways by caulking and sealing cracks and crevices in foundations, around exterior and interior water pipes.

Chemical controls consist of deterrents that can be applied as barriers or poisons in the form of residual sprays, powders, pellets, traps, and poison-loaded baits. It's important to remember that insecticides may also kill off cockroaches' natural predators, and chemical sprays may also aggravate allergies and asthma. The most common treatments include, from least to most toxic:

- natural pesticides like d-Limonene, orange peel extract, which both repels and kills insects, including roaches, by destroying the wax coating on their exoskeletons through which they breathe, and diatomaceous earth, or silica gel, which dehydrates them;
- boric acid–based powders and baits, which cause starvation and dehydration;
- sprays containing pyrethrins and other more toxic ingredients;
- bait stations containing any number of chemical poisons.

Fortunately, roaches respond well to the least toxic physical and chemical methods of prevention and elimination, so there's usually no need to threaten your own, your family's, or your pets' health with a lot of sprays and poisons, which is a counterproductive way to treat an allergy anyway.

In Summary

- There are nearly 40 cockroach species in Florida, but only a handful are considered indoor pests, namely the German, Australian, and American cockroaches.

- An estimated 26 percent of Americans exhibit allergic sensitivity to the German cockroach.
- Cockroach allergy is a significant factor in urban asthma cases in children, with more children allergic to cockroaches (37 percent) than to dust mites (35 percent) or cats (23 percent).
- Cockroach allergens stem from cockroach excrement, body secretions, cast skins, and carcasses.
- Cockroach allergens act directly on the respiratory and bronchial airway systems, causing inflammation and constriction.
- Sensitive individuals react to roach allergens at two to eight units (80 to 160 nanograms) per gram of dust. Research suggests that 11 percent of U.S. living rooms and 13 percent of U.S. kitchens exceed 2 U/g of cockroach allergens.
- People with chronic severe bronchial asthma, chronic rhinitis, sinus infections, and ear infections are most susceptible to cockroach allergy.
- Cockroach allergy symptoms can include itchy skin and irritated, scratchy throat, nose, or eyes. Persistent year-round asthma can also be a sign of cockroach allergy. Diagnosis is made at an allergist's office via skin test.
- Threefold treatment for cockroach allergy involves (1) prevention, through cleanliness and cockroach population control; (2) alleviation of symptoms with over-the-counter medications; and (3) immunotherapeutic mitigation with cockroach extracts, for which medical trials continue.
- Roach control takes two basic forms. Physical control involves maintaining cleanliness and proper food storage to reduce cockroach habitat. Chemical control involves the use of insecticides of varying toxicities to kill individual cockroaches and suppress population increase.
- Fortunately, cockroach allergy can be prevented or greatly alleviated with simple household measures and use of low toxicity chemical barriers and baits like boric acid or d-Limonene.

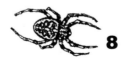

8

Along Came an Arachnid

The spider's touch, how exquisitely fine!
Feels at each thread, and lives along the line.

Alexander Pope

Arachnids are an extraordinarily diverse group of creatures, with more than 110,000 described species and possibly as many as a million. Besides their characteristic eight legs, they're also distinguished by a lack of antennae and a set of pointed, flexible appendages, called chelicerae, in place of mandibles (and from which their phylum, Chelicerata, which includes horseshoe crabs, gets its name). They use these chelicerae to grasp food or, in the case of spiders, whose chelicerae more closely resemble fangs, to inject venom.

All of these features combine in such diverse ways as to elicit a variety of usually unhappy responses from the humans who encounter them, often along the lines of swift movement in the opposite direction, or the fell swoop of a rolled-up newspaper.

Our abhorrence is unfortunate. Although a few arachnids can produce allergic responses in sensitive individuals, and some are, in fact, deadly, arachnids are ecologically vital creatures. Spiders actually eat more insects than do birds. And although people are more likely to squash a spider on sight, regardless of species, bees and wasps pose greater health risks than spiders, and dogs are more dangerous than either.

Nearly 5 million people are bitten by dogs each year, resulting in 800,000 visits to the hospital, compared with fewer than 5,000 cases of spider bites annually, of which only 10 percent require medical treatment.[1] Further, about 80 percent of injuries thought due to spider bites turn out to be attributed to punctures from things like thorns or bites from other insects.

In one perspective-setting four-year study, the Centers for Disease Control found that dog bites killed 20 people a year, and automobile collisions with deer killed 130 people. But there was not a single spider-related death during that time.[2] An estimated 25–35 percent of the population may be arachnaphobic.[3] But the number of people afraid of spiders far exceeds the number of people who will ever have a dangerous or allergenic encounter with one.

But spiders are only one of the eleven orders of arachnids, which also include scorpions, scorpion variants known as whip scorpions and pseudoscorpions, whip spiders, harvestmen (which despite appearances, are not spiders), and mites, the group to which ticks and chiggers belong.

Of all of them, allergic reactions to mite and tick bites are the most common. Spider bites typically act on the nervous system, muscles, tissue cells, and organs rather than on the immune system, and then usually only on creatures smaller than spiders. Recent research actually aims to put some of that toxicity to good use in treating everything from erectile dysfunction to cancer.[4]

But arachnaphobes care nothing of that, so let's go in for a closer look at the things that sit down beside us and frighten us all away.

Spiders—Allergy potential: Insignificant

Of the roughly 900 species of spiders in Florida, only five are considered venomous to humans. Actually, all spiders are venomous to some degree; that's how they kill their prey. But most people will never have a dangerous encounter with a spider, and in fact, most Floridians will probably only see about 10 percent of the spiders in Florida in their lifetime.[5]

Of the five spider species of possible concern to humans, four are widow spiders—the southern, northern, red, and brown widows. And the fifth is the inscrutable brown recluse.

Widow spiders (genus *Latrodectus*)

Widow spiders are all similar in size, appearance, behavior, and life cycle. About half an inch long with legs extended, they may vary a bit in color and habitat. But all widow females secure their pear-shaped egg sacs, containing a couple hundred eggs, in thick tangle webs with a conical area in the corner in which the spiders hide. All but the northern black widow breed year-round in Florida.

Widow spider bites don't feel like much, a pin prick perhaps, and

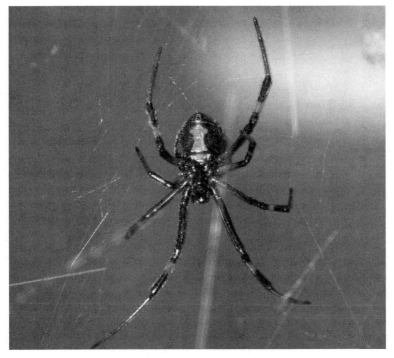

Young female black widow spider, just before the last molt; after the molt, she was totally black with no brown at all. (Photo by Joseph Berger, Bugwood.org. This work is licensed under a Creative Commons Attribution 3.0 License.)

despite the alarming descriptions of venom progression after a bite, citing things like muscle cramps and nausea, the truth is that not only are bites rare, but in the case of the dreaded black widow, they often don't even inject venom when they bite.

In near chastisement, a document about spider bites published by the California Poison Control System observes, "Spiders do not attack in herds. Spiders do not lie in wait and attack people. Spiders do not lift the covers at night and crawl into bed to bite people as they are sleeping. Some spiders can jump, but they are not intentionally jumping at humans to attack them. A spider generally bites a human because it was scared and bites to defend itself."[6]

And in fact, that is exactly how the rare spider bite occurs: a spider gets trapped against the skin and bites in self-defense.

In a thought-provoking study done in Australia in 2002, a country with more than its fair share of dangerous creatures, researchers studied 750 definite spider bite victims and learned the following:

- Significant effects occurred in just 6 percent (44) of the bite victims.
- Only 11 percent (6) of those people needed antivenin.
- No definite spider bites resulted in necrotic ulcers (areas of tissue death).
- Only 7 cases resulted in secondary infection, and more to our purposes here,
- No allergic reactions occurred.[7]

The study suggested that media attention to the rare fatal case fuels unsubstantiated arachnophobia and that the majority of spiders are not of "any medical significance."

In one classic case, a teacher brought a black widow spider with an egg sac to an elementary school classroom in Florida. When the egg sac hatched, hundreds of tiny black widows escaped into the classroom and students suddenly began experiencing flu-like symptoms, skin irritations, behavioral problems, and more, all of which were attributed to spider bites. The teacher was disciplined and the school fumigated. But experts point out that baby black widow chelicerae are far too weak to penetrate human skin, and the amount of venom that affects humans can only be produced by adult spiders.[8]

As a matter of fact, no deaths from widow spider envenomation have been reported in the United States since 1983, nor have any significant allergic responses.[9] So you can pretty much brush the widow spiders off your list of things to worry about.

Just don't reach into any dark corners in old dusty buildings. The rare reaction to widow spider venom isn't an allergic one, but a direct result of envenomation that, depending upon the age and physical condition of the victim, can be pretty painful.

Brown Recluse (*Loxosceles reclusa*)

The brown recluse is a species of great debate in Florida. Actual incidents of brown recluse bites are difficult to substantiate, and no established populations of these spiders have been found in Florida. That's not to say the spider doesn't occur in Florida or that its venom isn't dangerous.

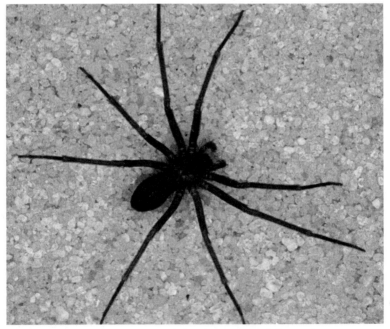

Brown recluse. (Photo courtesy of Florida Division of Plant Industry Archive, Florida Department of Agriculture and Consumer Services, Bugwood.org. Creative Commons Attribution 3.0 License.)

The venom of the brown recluse is very similar to snake venom. It's cytotoxic, or toxic to cells, and hemolytic, suppressing blood clotting, which causes necrosis, or tissue death. There is no antivenin for the bite of the brown recluse, so bites are treated with antibiotics and corticosteroids.[10]

But while the Florida Poison Control Network received nearly 300 reports of brown recluse bites in 2001, few were confirmed, and not a single brown recluse has ever been collected. Entomologist G. B. Edwards puts it more succinctly. On the basis of his own years of experience, and after reviewing the available data, he says, "It appears obvious to me that the chance of interaction between brown recluse spiders and people in Florida is close to nil."[11]

Other Notable Florida Spiders

While they produce no known allergies, several other Florida spiders are occasionally known to bite people, usually as a result of accidental encounters:

- Wandering spiders (family Ctenidae)—dark brown, half an inch long, with a broad tan stripe—prefer damp wooded areas. It's thought that many brown recluse bite reports may actually be bites from the Florida wandering spider.[12]
- Sac spiders (family Cheiracanthiumare) are small yellowish spiders common in fields and agricultural areas. They make nests of rolled-up leaves. Their bites are painful and can produce nausea, muscle pain, and minor tissue necrosis around the bite area.
- Giant crab spiders (family Sparassidae) can be the size of coffee saucers, with the male huntsman spider's legs spanning five inches. They're disconcertingly fast, necessarily so to catch their preferred prey of cockroaches and silverfish. When trapped, they can give a pretty nasty bite that will swell for a few days.
- Orbweavers (family Nephilidae) can also be huge, two to three inches in diameter, and often brilliantly colored. They live outdoors and are more of an issue for hikers who inadvertently stumble into one of their huge webs.

- Wolf spiders (family Lycosidaeare) are impressive hairy arachnids that don't spin webs, but fleetly chase prey. They are among the most diverse and abundant spiders in the world, and there are several species in Florida.
- Tarantulas (family Theraphosidaeare) are non-native, although the Mexican red rump tarantula has become established in some parts of Florida as a result of the exotic pet trade. They can be venomous to humans, but are usually reluctant to bite, and no allergic or fatal reactions have been reported. Tarantula body hairs apparently pose a bigger problem for people, producing an itching similar to that encountered by contact with fiberglass.[13]

Spider Habitat

Widow spiders typically shelter in a corner of their irregular tangled webs in quiet, undisturbed areas, often near the ground. The best time to locate them is at night, with a flashlight. They can usually be found in small crevices, eaves, beneath wooden outdoor furniture, under trailers, and in piles of wood, bricks, or concrete blocks. The knowledge that one usually has to go to such great lengths to even find a widow spider should be reassuring.[14]

The chance of seeing a brown recluse is even more remote. Their indoor habitat, however, includes closets, neglected piles of clothing, crawl spaces, window wells, and baseboard cracks and crevices.

Most other spider species occur as expected—outdoors in places conducive to their insect prey, in gardens, in hidden areas in and around a home, and often in piles of debris or clutter.

Recognizing and Treating Spider Bites

A spider bite may not be noticed right away, especially one from a widow spider, until the bite area becomes painful. Widow spider venom contains neurotoxic proteins that spread through the lymphatic system and, depending on the amount of venom injected, can produce a massive release of neurotransmitters and commensurate symptoms of pain and muscle tightness.

While most spider bites aren't dangerous, if a widow spider or a brown recluse bite is suspected, it's a good idea to get prompt medical attention. Identification of the spider that causes a bite is important in treating the injury, and the best way to get a positive ID is to collect the suspected culprit, in whatever shape it remains after delivering a bite, and preserve it in a container with rubbing alcohol.[15]

Widow bites are more dangerous to young children and the elderly, but the symptoms of a widow bite can be uncomfortable for anyone and may include headache, lethargy, nausea, shortness of breath, intense muscle pain, and rigidity of abdomen and legs. An injection of calcium gluconate can relieve the pain if antivenin is not available. While a rash may sometimes develop, the greater risk of allergic reaction is to the horse-serum antivenin, so there is some argument about the use of antivenin in treating bites in non-risk populations.[16]

Brown recluse bites, if they can even be identified, may go completely unnoticed and require absolutely no care, or may result in a mild to severe localized necrotic reaction at the site of the bite, which heals slowly. Capturing a suspected brown recluse is helpful to those providing treatment, since there is no antivenin but other treatments can control symptoms and limit tissue damage. Sac spider bite reactions are more recognizably allergenic in nature, initially painful, and accompanied by redness, itching, and swelling. They can produce small necrotic wounds, but usually heal quickly. Ice usually helps relieve symptoms.[17]

For all types of spider bites, general wound treatment consists of washing the bite area, calming the bite victim, and consulting a doctor as soon as possible, unless you're confident with your spider ID.

Spider Control

Spiders can be difficult to control chemically, since little of their body comes into contact with insecticidal sprays or powders, and egg sacs are usually protected from both as well.

Indoors, mechanical controls like sweeping and vacuuming regularly can be very effective, especially along normally undisturbed areas like baseboards, crevices, and behind and under furniture to remove webs and egg sacs and potential spider prey.[18] Tarantulas have poor eyesight, and control can be a matter of sweeping one into a dustbin and depositing it outside.

To reduce incoming populations of spiders, keep woodpiles away from a home, check carefully for spiders when bringing wood or plants inside, and clear debris regularly from around home foundations.

Outdoor Protection

We're "Big Stick" hikers, especially in close brush and thickly forested areas, using either a walking stick or a large branch to sweep ahead of us as we hike. Webs can be almost impossible to see depending on lighting. Avoid reaching blindly and bare-handed into holes, brush, or enclosed areas.

Wear gloves when gardening, and avoid loose-fitting clothing that allows spiders and other small, probably unwelcome creatures to inadvertently hitch a ride. Try to suppress the "swatting" response. Move smoothly and intentionally to sweep any intruder away gently, rather than pressing it against you with a heavy-handed whack, which provokes a stinging or biting response from most stinging and biting creatures.

All of these measures, however, will simply reduce chance encounters with spiders, not eliminate them, because spiders are, by their nature, nearly everywhere we like to be. Fortunately, while the rare spider bite can be painful, allergic responses are uncommon.

Scorpions (order Scorpiones)—Allergy potential: Insignificant

Scorpions are an ancient species of arachnid, virtually unchanged for millennia. Like spiders, they have eight legs, as well as a characteristic stinger and a set of pinchers that they use far more often than the stinger.

Florida is home to just three scorpion species, ranging in size from one to four inches in length:

- Florida bark scorpion, our largest species, also known as the slender brown scorpion

- Guiana striped scorpion, which confines itself to Collier, Miami-Dade, and Monroe counties
- Hentz striped, the smallest and most common species[19]

Most local poison control centers and much medical literature assure in consistent, nearly verbatim language that "Florida scorpions are NOT venomous." Actually, only pseudoscorpions like whip scorpions (also known as vinegaroons for their distinctive and off-putting chemical defense), wind spiders, and whip spiders are truly venomless; they vaguely resemble scorpions, and none bear stingers.

The statement should actually read, "Florida scorpions are not venomous to humans." Like spiders, true scorpions can't live without their venom, and their curled anterior stinger is an efficient venom delivery system. While stings may be painful, scorpion venom is a neurotoxin that produces few dermatologic effects beyond redness and swelling at the sting site.[20]

There is some evidence of cross-reactivity to scorpion venom in those who have had previous exposure, but the American Academy of Allergy, Asthma and Immunology (AAAAI) reports that scorpions rarely cause allergic reactions.[21] And it's hard to get stung by a scorpion in the first place. They normally live outdoors, are mostly active at night, and don't sting unprovoked. They go out of their way to avoid problems with anything larger than themselves, and with just a few precautions on the human end, it's pretty easy to accommodate them.

Scorpion Habitat

Scorpions shelter under boards, woodpiles, and debris. In Florida, they may occur in and around newly built homes. But they prefer and thrive in the outdoors where they dine on insects, spiders, and other small creatures.[22]

Scorpions are nocturnal. As a matter of fact, one of the best ways to spot scorpions is to use a portable black light at night and look for their characteristic fluorescent glow. Encounters are almost always accidental, usually the result of reaching blindly into dark spaces, including utility areas, firewood piles, attics, or crawl spaces.

Treating Scorpion Bites

Scorpion bites should be cleaned with soap and water. Ice packs can help relieve pain and swelling, but no other care is usually indicated.

Scorpion Control

Scorpion control is usually just a matter of eliminating or reducing scorpion habitat and using care when working in areas where scorpions might naturally occur. And there are some things homeowners can do to discourage scorpions.

- Trim overhanging branches away from walls and roof areas.
- Use cement blocks or bricks to elevate trash cans and firewood.
- Use gloves when handling firewood, and only bring it indoors when ready to use it.
- Keep window screens and weather stripping in good repair.
- Caulk cracks around windows or doors.

Suspected scorpion infestations can be treated with residual pesticides, although this is usually unnecessary. Removing scorpions indoors is often just a matter of scooping them up in a dustpan and depositing them outside. Outdoors, if you're of a farmyard sort of mind, ducks and chickens are good biological controls for reducing scorpion populations.

Outdoor Protection

Common sense goes a long way in protecting against scorpion stings.

- Avoid going barefoot, especially around water sources or preferred scorpion habitat like woodpiles and yard debris.
- When camping or hiking, shake out shoes and check clothing and sleeping bags carefully before wearing or using, especially items that have been left on the ground.
- Wear long sleeves and pants when hiking or camping in areas where scorpions may be common.
- Don't sit on old logs or reach into dark holes, brush, or debris piles.[23]

Mites and Ticks (order Acari)—Allergy potential: High

Spiders can be scary because they're leggy and visible. Scorpions look like alien invaders. But mites are the real skeletons in the arachnid closet, responsible for a host of problems, from costly agricultural and horticultural damage to human ills ranging from severe allergies to fatal diseases.

Mites and ticks are actually one and the same creature. Ticks are simply giant mites, and the whole collective is cataloged within the order Acari. Mites are the most abundant and diverse of the arachnids and among the oldest of all terrestrial creatures, with a lineage dating back 400 million years.[24] Although 45,000 species have been described, that may be only about 5 percent of the actual number of species of mites on earth.

They live nearly everywhere, from deserts to the Arctic, from boreal forests to deep sea trenches, and on nearly every living thing. Many species have symbiotic relationships with their hosts, including humans, who are populated by hair follicle mites living contentedly in the universe of our eyebrows and eyelashes.

Mites have sucking mouthparts for taking in liquid food of either a plant or animal nature. In the absence of the usual animal host, mites will often latch onto the nearest human. And there are plenty of mites that dine solely on humans. In most cases, bites can be painful, itchy, and cause anything from rashes to difficulty breathing. Additionally, the skins and feces of mites, like those of cockroaches, can cause inflammation and contraction of the airways.

Some common Florida mites that can attack humans include

- bird mites, common in bird-infested buildings;
- insect mites, especially the straw itch mite, which can cause severe dermatitis;
- rodent mites, which can also cause severe dermatitis as well as secondary infections from scratching;
- scabies mites, also known as human itch mites;
- house dust mites, of enormous significance nationwide;
- chiggers, or red bugs, whose saliva can trigger severe dermatitis; and
- ticks.

The principal culprit in most tick bite reactions is due to a sensitivity to tick saliva. One theory is that histamine-binding proteins in the saliva of biting arthropods like mites and ticks, injected during the blood-feeding process, can lower blood pressure, dilate capillaries, and increase blood flow, triggering inflammation and allergy.[25]

The Mighty Mite

Mites have short, quick life cycles of one to four weeks from egg to larvae to nymph to adult, resulting in abundant populations under the right conditions.[26]

Some mites, like bird and rodent mites, are accidental pests caused by infestations of birds or rodents in buildings. While these animal mites usually stick to their traditional menu, they can and will bite humans with itchy results. Scratching bites can also result in secondary infections.

The straw itch mite is a nightmarish-looking creature (or would be if you could see it), a living pincushion of tiny hairs and hooks. Considered something of a beneficial insect, it makes its living on alfalfa, barley, and related grasses, preying on resident grain moths and furniture beetles. As tiny as the straw itch mite is—about $1/32$ inch after eating, and undetectable to the human eye between meals—the female can store up to 300 eggs in her body and give live birth to an invisible swarm that can breed within a week.

One to several hundred bites can occur on people or animals, although neither may notice for up to a day, after which a dermatitis consisting of red welts with a small white pustule at the center may occur. In severe cases, the bites can cause infection, fever, vomiting, and joint pain, plus secondary infection from scratching open the pustules. Itching can last a week or more, and it will be another few weeks before the welts abate.[27]

Scabies Mite

Scabies mites have evolved to infect almost all mammals, including pets, livestock, and wildlife. The mite that literally makes our skin crawl is also known as the human itch mite, and it has been tormenting humans since there have been humans to torment. Infinitesimal at $1/64$ inch and looking like some alien hot air balloon, the scabies mite essentially causes human mange when the female burrows under folds of skin to lay eggs. There, nymphs hatch and develop, burrowing further into the skin.

Severe itching is usually the main symptom of scabies. It's common in crowded environments and especially among school children, since it can be easily transmitted by direct contact and by sharing beds and clothing. Additionally, dog scabies can and often do infect humans.

Extensive rashes develop following sensitization to subsequent bites, starting around the armpits, wrists, waist, neck, and back of calves, and eventually spreading across the body, beyond the actual site of infestation.

House Dust Mite

The scourge of homes everywhere, the house dust mite causes allergies the same way cockroaches do, through excretions, the primary allergenic trigger, as well as secretions and their cast-off molted skins. About 4 percent of all humans are thought to have allergies caused by dust mites. Of all the arachnids, the house dust mite is the most significant in terms of allergies worldwide.

In an interesting twist, house dust mites function as something of a human cleaning crew, feasting on our own shed skin particles, which we slough off at the rate of about five grams a week. One gram of our dermal detritus, it has been estimated, can feed thousands of mites for months. This is manna from heaven for invisible hoards that produce a new generation every three weeks.[28]

And in return, dust mites make us itch, cough, and gasp for air. Inhaled mite allergens trigger IgG, IgE, and IgA antibodies in allergic individuals, producing symptoms of eczema and asthma, often in a delayed response anywhere from 2 to 12 hours after exposure.

Thanks to our humid climate and relatively stable temperatures, dust mites have found a particularly suitable environment in Florida.[29] They occur in all homes and are particularly fond of carpets and drapes. They're also common in schools and daycare centers. In one study of 20 daycare facilities in Tampa alone, 40 percent had levels of mite allergens exceeding those associated with sensitization.[30]

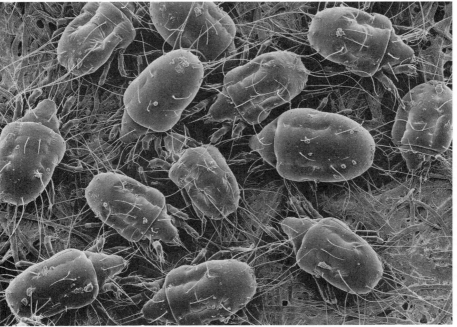

House dust mites, magnified. (Photo by Eric Erbe, USDA.)

Mite Habitat

"Su casa es mi casa" might be the mite motto. Human mites tend to inhabit human habitats. Carpeting, heavy curtains, fabric-covered furniture, linens, and pillows are the favorite haunts of dust mites. Scabies mites can be found on linens and clothing. Mites of other animals can get on humans from infestations of the animals in households and buildings.

Treating Mite Bites

Bites should be washed and antiseptic applied. Local anesthetics and antihistamines can be applied to ease irritation and itching. If severe dermatitis occurs from mite bites, a dermatologist should be consulted. Outdoor precautions include avoiding grassy areas and washing with plenty of soap and water after being in such areas.

Controlling Mites

Mite infestations from mite hosts like birds or rodents can be controlled by eliminating rodent nests and bird roosting areas and using residual crack and crevice treatments to kill mites employing those pathways. Most mites cannot live more than 24 hours off their host, so eliminating host infestations can be the most effective way to deal with bird, rodent, and insect mites.[31]

Outdoors, control can be seasonally achieved, as mite populations tend to decrease in cold weather. Removal of straw, hay, grain, or wood piles can be helpful in eliminating the straw itch mite. To control scabies mites, consult a physician, and if scabies transmission is thought to be from an infected pet, visit a veterinarian for appropriate treatment for the animal.

House mite infestations can be confirmed with diagnostic tests like Acarex, which actually looks for the presence of house dust mite feces in dust samples.[32] Controlling house mites can be an elaborate process that includes

- frequent washing of bedding and curtains in hot water (130F);
- regular vacuuming with a HEPA-equipped machine;
- using HEPA air cleaners and air filters for air-conditioning and heating units;
- removal of carpeting;
- dust control through the use of nonfibrous bedding or mattress covers, synthetic pillows, and nylon or cotton cellulose blankets;
- use of ozone air purifiers;
- decreasing humidity with a dehumidifier; and
- Acaricide treatments.

While routine vacuuming and changing linens are among the prescribed treatments for dust mite reduction, this temporarily increases mite allergen levels in the air. For that reason, water-filtered vacuums are sometimes recommended. Regular vacuuming and environmental control are usually the best preventatives.

Chemical controls are limited, with only two nonpesticide products, Acarosan and Allergy Control Solution, both containing benzyl benzoate and tannic acid as their active ingredients, showing significant effectiveness against mites. Pyrethrins have also proven helpful, although regular preventative measures appear to be the most effective control.

Chiggers

Chiggers, also known as "jiggers" and "red bugs," are a type of mite larvae with an unfortunate ability to cause horrendously itchy red welts wherever they bite. In some parts of the world, they can transmit typhus. But in Florida, they only spread itching and possibly secondary infections from the relentless scratching of victims.

Whereas cold weather can reduce chigger populations in more continental climates, in Florida, chiggers are active year-round, producing crops of minute, practically invisible ($1/50$ inch long) six-legged reddish parasitic larvae. Chiggers crawl about until they find suitable hosts, including mammals, birds, reptiles, or amphibians.

After latching on, they inject an enzyme that dissolves tissues into the liquefied diet they require. Humans are considered "accidental" hosts. They're not aiming for us; we just stumble into their paths. Chiggers on humans usually detach or die within a few hours, since our immune response to their bite disables them.[33]

That doesn't make the experience any less harrowing. Lilian Norris of Tampa, an active outdoorswoman, had a memorable encounter with chiggers during a fall camping trip to Ocala National Forest.

After camping the first night under some large oaks, Norris and her companion retreated into a cabin when an unexpected and rainy cold front came through.

We had to gather our bedding and clothes that we had previously left in our tent. So we tromped out into the dark with a flashlight and umbrella to retrieve our belongings. The wet ground was sparse, mainly covered with oak leaves, but there were some areas of low grasses and weeds. Our shoes and ankle socks became moist as we walked. Due to the drop in temperature and our failure to pack sufficient clothes for cooler weather, we left our socks on our cold feet and slipped into our sleeping bags.

The next morning, the campers awoke to find their feet and ankles covered with hundreds of red blistery, itchy pustules.

> Even though our feet initially looked similar, I suffered a worse reaction to these bites than my friend. My bites worsened in 24–48 hours from the time I first noticed them, getting larger and itchier. The bites were like nothing I experienced before—similar to ant bites, but with pustules much, much larger on top of big red welts. I had so many bites that my feet and ankles swelled.

Norris had to go barefoot or wear loose slippers for more than a week. "Calamine lotion definitely helped," she said. "But it still didn't take away the intense, crazy itch."

Norris's is a textbook chigger encounter. Chiggers have been described as simply "bags of water"[34] that require high humidity and moisture to survive—the exact habitat where Norris and her friend first pitched their tent. Chiggers wait on the ground or along grass blades until, stimulated by movement and the carbon dioxide of a potential host, they move quickly to attach to the body within closest reach.

They favor areas constricted by clothing or where flesh is thin, tender, or has folds, which usually means around the ankles, waist, knees, groin, or armpits. Itching usually starts within four to eight hours of bites, and the longer chiggers are attached, as in Norris's overnight situation, the larger the welts and the greater the itching.

As Norris discovered, chigger bites can cause severe allergic responses, and reactions can vary greatly between individuals. Old wives' tales aside, however, chiggers do not embed themselves in the skin. The itchy welts produced by chigger bites can last up to two weeks and are thought to be caused by the digestive enzyme that chiggers inject to make their meals palatable.

Chigger Habitat

Because of their need for moisture and humidity, chiggers (and ticks) prefer thick vegetation like overgrown, undisturbed areas along forest edges, power line corridors, berry patches, shrubby and weedy areas, and anywhere rodents, reptiles, and other appropriate hosts are common.[35] They can also occur in home lawns if hosts are readily available and other conditions are supportive.

Treating Chigger Bites

A hot, soapy bath or shower that includes a couple of good latherings easily removes chiggers from the skin and kills them, and this is always recommended after hiking or working in chigger habitat. Welts may still appear, since symptoms take a few hours to kick in, but prompt showering or bathing should greatly reduce problems.

Apply antiseptic to any welts that do appear, and use standard over-the-counter anti-itch treatments like hydrocortisone, calamine lotion, and antihistamine creams prepared with lidocaine or benzocaine to help relieve itching.

Some home remedies reputed to help reduce itching include rubbing a paste of meat tenderizer (papain, without salt) or baking soda onto welts, or sponging them with vinegar. Alison Shephard of Clearwater swears by "flowers of sulphur," which she learned about during her work as a drafter on a field survey crew.

"Our party chief . . . had a baggie of a fine pale yellow powder he called flowers of sulphur. We all just took about a quarter teaspoon, as I remember, each morning the first week. After establishing a level of it in our blood, we'd take it less often. We took it with breakfast before going out into chigger territory. Chiggers were not a problem."

She thinks it may have kept off other bugs as well, and she may be right. Elemental sulphur, which can be purchased in most drugstores, has been used for years as an insect repellent.

It's also important to keep affected areas clean and avoid scratching welts, which can cause secondary infection from opened wounds. Report any unusual reactions including fever, difficulty breathing, or infection to a doctor.

Chigger Control

A good way to identify chigger populations in a yard is to place a piece of black cardboard edgewise in the ground. Chiggers will climb to the top, where they'll appear as tiny yellow or pinkish dots moving across the cardboard. The best way to reduce chigger infestations in residential areas is to keep brush cleared and grass closely mown.

Several insecticides will treat against chiggers. Attempts to reduce populations of reptiles, amphibians, and small mammals that serve as hosts for chiggers can also help, but may be impractical as well as counterproductive, since these creatures can serve as biological controls for other undesirable insects and animals. However, securing trash cans and reducing other inadvertent feeding areas created by rotting fruit or discarded seed can help reduce common chigger hosts like rats, possums, or raccoons.

Outdoor Protection

Commercially available repellents that contain any combination of permethrin, diethyl toluamide, dimethyl phthalate, dimethyl carbate, ethyl hexanediol, and benzyl benzoate are effective against chigger bites as well as against mosquitoes and other insects. Repellents can last for several hours or days if clothing is saturated by spraying or soaking.[36] Apply skin repellents to legs, ankles, waist, and wrists. Common dusting sulfur can also be effective as a skin-based repellent.

Wearing protective and properly fitted clothing is also important. Avoid clothing that is too tight or too loose and dragging on the ground. Also avoid sitting or lying on bare ground when working outdoors, camping, or picnicking in areas where chiggers may be a problem, and don't leave clothing on the ground.

Keep the problem in perspective, too. Lilian Norris notes that she camped in Ocala many times before and after her unfortunate chigger encounter, and never before or since has she suffered anything similar to the severe reaction she had that one fall.

"The experience has not hindered my passion for the outdoors," she says. "But it has made me be a little more careful and enlightened. I will always change all my clothing before going to bed after visiting a wild area, now that I know that chigger larvae could still be present."

The Terrible Tick

The tick is the bloodthirsty giant of the mite family. Whereas dust mites are too small to see, ticks can vary in size from the tiny deer tick, which is no bigger than a grain of pepper, to the quarter-inch whitish-green blob of an engorged dog tick.

The most common ticks in Florida are the American and the brown dog ticks. The deer tick isn't that abundant. But the lone star tick and the Gulf Coast tick are, and they can wreak significant health havoc on hikers and outdoors enthusiasts.

Ticks can be hard or soft bodied. Unable to fly or jump, ticks lie in wait for a host on the hoof. Lab studies have shown they can survive for up to three years without a meal. When they do detect motion, they latch onto passing mammals—wildlife, domestic pets, or people—sometimes by the dozens, with a fierce tenacity and the single-minded goal of a blood meal.

While tick bites aren't painful, their saliva can cause allergic reactions and, more problematically, can also transmit a variety of diseases via viruses, bacteria, or parasites. Illnesses commonly associated with tick bites include

- Lyme disease, from the bite of the deer tick;
- Rocky Mountain spotted fever, with 19 cases reported in Florida in 2008, mostly in northern and central counties;[37]
- human monocytic ehrlichiosis (HME) and human granulo-cytotropic anaplasmosis (HGA), bacterial diseases only rarely found in Florida, occurring in the north and central parts of the state;[38]
- southern tick-associated rash illness (STARI), similar to Lyme disease, thought to be transmitted by the lone star tick;[39]
- babesiosis, not considered a health threat in Florida;[40]
- Rickettsia parkeri, occurring in Florida where it is transmitted by the Gulf Coast tick and possibly the lone star tick;[41]
- tularemia, an ulcerative and lymphatic illness; and
- tick paralysis, fortunately a rare and quickly reversible condi-

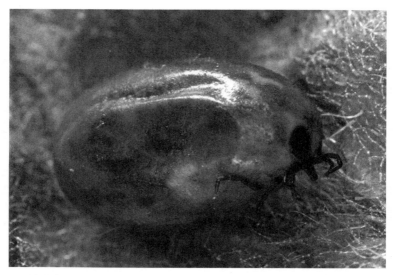

An adult female blacklegged tick, engorged after a blood meal, rests on a leaf. (Photo by Scott Bauer, USDA Agricultural Research Service.)

tion (by removal of the tick), known to occur in dogs and in children, where it is sometimes misdiagnosed as Guillain-Barre syndrome.[42]

Tick-bite Allergy or Tick-borne Disease?

Because of the severity of some of these illnesses, it is important to be able to distinguish between an allergic reaction to a tick bite and a potentially more serious response and to get the appropriate medical care. An allergic response is characterized by

1. rashes or swelling that remain localized at bite sites;
2. bite marks that don't exceed two inches in diameter; and
3. bite marks that disappear within a few days.[43]

More serious tick-borne illnesses are usually characterized by lethargy, fever, and muscle aches. According to the Florida Department of Health, some of the more common serious illnesses have fairly specific symptoms:

- Lyme disease is often identified by a "bull's eye" rash that occurs in 60–80 percent of victims between 3 and 30 days after the bite of an infected tick. The rash can occur at the site of the bite or anywhere else on the body. Other symptoms include headache, chills, fatigue, stiff neck, or muscle aches.
- HME and HGA symptoms are often so mild that people don't go to the doctor. Those who do become ill may experience symptoms 5 to 10 days after a bite, including fever, headache, fatigue, and muscle aches. Children often develop a rash, while adults usually don't. Removing attached ticks within 24 hours significantly reduces the chance of developing this potentially fatal disease.
- Rocky Mountain spotted fever produces a characteristic red rash within 2 to 5 days after the onset of a fever that is first detected on the wrists and ankles. The rash progresses systematically through the palms, soles, arms, legs, and trunk. Muscle aches, lack of appetite, and diarrhea are also common. Some people will have no rash at all. The disease can be treated with antibiotics and prevented by prompt removal of any attached ticks, since studies have shown ticks need to be attached for 6 to 20 hours to transmit the illness.
- STARI can be confused with Lyme disease because it produces an almost identical "bull's eye" rash that develops about a week after a bite and then expands outward from the bite area. Fever, lethargy, headaches, and joint pain are also symptoms, but STARI does not produce the chronic arthritis and neurological symptoms that Lyme disease can cause. STARI is treated with antibiotics.

A Helpful Allergy

In an interesting twist, those predisposed to tick bite allergy may actually be somewhat protected against more serious illnesses like Lyme disease. Researchers in New England found that those who had "persistent itch and local swelling" in response to tick bites were less likely to acquire Lyme disease.[44]

"The acquisition of Lyme disease increased from 15 percent to 25 percent to 31 percent among participants who reported no itch, one episode of tick-associated itch, and two reports of itch, respectively," the researchers noted.

They theorize that itching provides a helpful early sign of tick bites and spurs prompt removal of ticks before any disease can be transmitted. They further speculated, "Additional inflammatory reaction to tick salivary proteins also may help prevent transmission."

Delayed Anaphylaxis

If your blood type is other than A or AB, another recent study has found an amazing allergic response to some tick bites: delayed anaphylaxis when eating certain meats. In a report originally hailing from Australia but since confirmed by University of Virginia researchers, individuals who had been bitten by "seed" ticks—the six-legged tiny larval young of adult ticks—experienced severe anaphylactic reactions 3 to 6 hours after eating beef, pork, or lamb.[45]

Patients first experienced an increasingly intensifying itching that spread across the skin's outer and deeper layers, and escalated to swelling, intestinal distress, and finally symptoms of anaphylaxis. Researchers narrowed the culprit of the delayed anaphylaxis to an IgE antibody that binds to a sugar molecule known as alpha-gal. The discovery of this antibody throws the current understanding of how allergies occur into disarray.

"Today's textbooks tell us that allergic reactions are caused by proteins in food, pollen, dander, and venom," the study's lead author, Dr. Scott Commins, is quoted as saying in news reports about the discovery. "They are not supposed to be caused by sugars like alpha-gal."

Early studies suggest all type of ticks—dog ticks, deer ticks, lone star ticks, and others—can trigger this reaction, which Commins says many people may have experienced without recognizing it.

A few unique aspects of "delayed anaphylaxis" make a clearer understanding of it challenging:

- People with A or AB type blood seem protected from developing IgE antibody to alpha-gal.
- Skin prick tests are ineffective at identifying the tick-induced red meat allergy.

- Most patients begin experiencing symptoms only in adult-hood.

In the meantime, Dr. Commins recommends the usual treatment to offset chances of tick-borne illness or allergy: prompt removal of ticks.

Tick Habitat

Tick habitats vary somewhat between species. Generally, though, all ticks dwell in areas where they can come into contact with their desired host.[46] With the exception of the forest-dwelling lone star tick, this means grassy and brushy areas along forest edges. Because

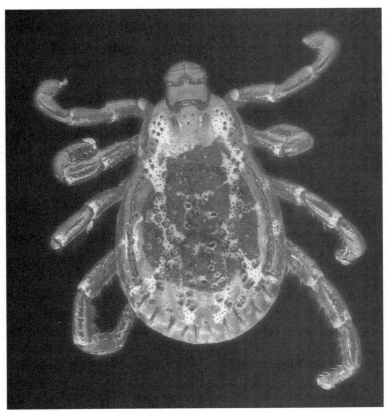

American dog tick. (Photo by Susan Ellis, USDA APHIS PPQ, Bugwood.org. This work is licensed under a Creative Commons Attribution 3.0 License.)

of heat and moisture needs, ticks are rarely found in lawns beyond a few feet from the edge of wooded areas.

American dog ticks live in old-field environments, along trails and paths, in pastures, and along the wooded margins of forests. An unwitting hiker, walking along a trail on a forest edge, can easily collect adult American dog, lone star, and deer ticks on a single hike.

In suburban Florida settings, the American dog tick can be found in vacant lots and overgrown yards and right of ways. And in some cases, the brown dog tick has adapted to live indoors, completing its entire life cycle for generations entirely on domestic dogs, causing problems in kennels and homes.

Treating Tick Bites

Attached ticks should be removed right away with a pair of fine-tipped tweezers or a commercial tick removal tool. Do not use petroleum jelly, lit or hot matches, or nail polish to remove ticks. The proper removal technique is to grasp the tick as close to the surface of the skin as possible and pull upward, steadily and evenly. Avoid squeezing or crushing a tick while removing it, to prevent the risk of expressing infectious fluids or breaking off its mouth parts in the skin.

After the tick is removed, wash and disinfect the bite site and wash hands well with soap and water. The tick may be saved in a dated plastic bag for identification, especially useful if symptoms develop later on.

Tick Control

The best way to control ticks around a home or yard is to keep grass closely cut and well maintained and to create tick-free landscaping, especially near wooded areas.[47]

- Keep yards free of debris like dead leaves and grass clippings.
- Keep flowerbeds dry.
- Keep bushes and shrubs trimmed, especially near paths and walkways.
- Create a three-foot gravel or mulch barrier to separate your lawn from any wooded areas, a helpful technique around children's play areas, birdfeeders, and woodpiles as well.

Chemical controls that treat the home, yard, and pets can be effective for tick infestations. Keep dogs and cats regularly treated with appropriate medications to prevent tick infestation, but always regularly examine pets for ticks, especially during the summer months, and promptly remove any that are found.

Residual sprays and dusts, lightly used as spot treatments, can be helpful in controlling light infestations of ticks, indoors and out. Take the usual precautions when using any sprays around pets or people, and do not treat pets with household pesticides. Outdoors, spray applications around foundations, by roadsides, trails, and paths used by people and pets.

Outdoor Protection

The best way to stay safe from ticks outdoors is to stay away from places ticks lie in wait, like forest edges, and grassy, brush-filled areas. For those understandably unwilling to give up their time in our great outdoors, though, several helpful measures can be taken.[48]

- Apply appropriate repellents, those usually containing DEET, picaridin, or IR3535, to skin and clothing to inhibit tick attacks.
- Wear light-colored clothing so that ticks can be seen more easily.
- "Blouse" pant legs—tuck them inside socks or boots when hiking—to help prevent ticks from crawling up inside loose pant legs.
- Stick to the center of trails, away from brush-filled or grassy edges.
- Perform personal tick checks and examine hiking companions after venturing into likely tick areas.
- Promptly remove any attached ticks.

In Summary

- Spiders, scorpions, mites, and ticks are all arachnids.
- Despite occasionally painful encounters, neither spiders nor scorpions usually cause allergies or serious injury.
- Mites, including ticks and chiggers, pose the most significant allergenic and health threat among arachnids.

- Histamine-binding proteins in the saliva of ticks, mites, and chiggers produce allergic responses in sensitive individuals.
- Dust mite allergy is one of the most widespread allergies, thought to be caused by inhalation of dust mite feces and other secretions.
- Dust mites can be controlled by regular vacuuming, washing linens in hot water, and reducing dust mite habitat, such as heavy drapes and rugs.
- Chiggers are a type of mite larvae whose bites can cause severe itchy red welts and secondary infections from scratching.
- Avoid chiggers by dressing properly when outdoors, staying off the ground in areas where chiggers may be present, and taking hot, soapy showers or baths promptly after possible contact.
- Ticks can transmit several different kinds of diseases, in addition to producing allergic reactions.
- An allergic response to a tick bite is characterized by limited rashes less than two inches in diameter that typically disappear within a few days.
- More serious tick-borne illnesses may be characterized by lethargy, fever, and muscle aches.
- Tick bite allergy may protect against more serious illnesses like Lyme disease, possibly because the itching response leads to prompt removal of ticks.
- A recently discovered tick-induced condition, "delayed anaphylaxis," is a cross-reactive allergy to beef, pork, or lamb in certain individuals who have been bitten by larval "seed" ticks.
- Tick-related illnesses and allergies can be ameliorated by conducting frequent tick checks when working or playing in suspected tick habitats and by prompt removal of ticks with a fine set of tweezers or other tick removal tool.

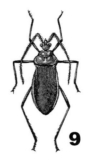

9

Assorted Arthropoda

insects have their own point of view about civilization
a man thinks he amounts to a great deal but to a flea or a mosquito
a human being is merely something good to eat

Don Marquis, *Archy's Maxims*

One might hope the tidy groups of insects previously presented would be the sum of small terrors in Florida. However, there are several other groups of stinging and biting arthropods in Florida that can also cause allergic responses. Most of these creatures, with the exception of caterpillars, bite rather than sting, and few, if any, are as problematic as Hymenoptera.[1] Only the biting flies come close.

Allergy potential varies with degree of exposure. Those whose work requires regular handling of insects like mealworms, locusts, or blowflies, for examples, or those exposed to mites or beetles in bakeries or similar environments can develop allergies known as baker's or grocer's itch.[2] Most of the insects and bugs in this section, however, typically produce allergies along the lines of some form of dermatitis.

We'll start our look at the miscellaneous stinging and biting arthropods in Florida with the "true bugs."

The True Bugs (order Hemiptera)

While we often interchangeably refer to insects as "bugs," the true bugs of the Hemiptera, which means "half wing," are physically distinct among arthropods. In addition to the bisected forewing from which they get their scientific name, all true bugs have wings that fold flat over the back, sucking and piercing mouth parts, and "stink" glands near the base of the middle pair of legs.

There are about 800 species of true bugs in Florida. The largest is the four-inch-long giant water bug, which makes horrific headlines when swarms periodically descend on shopping center parking lots. Nicknamed the "toe biter" for the rare but painful encounters with them waders may experience, the giant water bug prefers minnows and tadpoles and, appearances aside, is not a threat to people.

The assassin bug, however, is another story.

Assassin bugs (family Reduviidae)—Allergy potential: Moderate

Assassin bugs inflict a bite that is not only painful but also potentially dangerous. They can cause allergic reactions as well as localized injury that can take months to heal.[3] Fortunately, only a couple of the 65 or so species of assassin bugs in Florida are problematic, namely, the wheel bug and the cone-nose bug, and encounters with either are infrequent.

Named for their aggressive hunting style, assassin bugs are usually beneficial insects in Florida gardens. They lie in wait for smaller prey like caterpillars, beetles, aphids, and leafhoppers, into which they inject paralytic venom that turns prey into a liquefied meal. The wheel bug is capped by a spiky protrusion behind its head that looks quite like a gear wheel.

Water bug and wheel bug bites usually occur accidentally, either through inadvertent contact while wading, in the case of the water bugs, or through handling. Sometimes wheel bugs are encountered while gardening or hiking, and the bugs will bite if trapped against the skin. Orchard workers can be bitten by the bugs when working among trees.[4] Beyond the redness and swelling of urticaria and some residual tenderness, few other allergic responses to wheel bug bites have been reported.

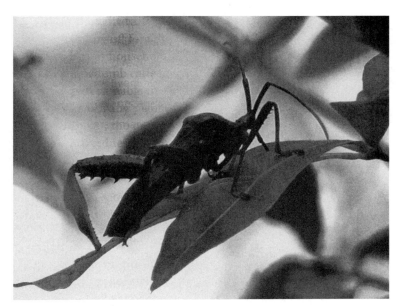

Assassin bug. (Photo by Theresa Willingham.)

Treatment consists of the usual protocol.

- Wash the bite area and apply antiseptic, especially after wading or working in or around soil.
- Standard, over-the-counter pain relievers like aspirin, acetaminophen, or ibuprofen can help reduce pain or discomfort.
- Calamine lotion or topical corticosteroids can help reduce swelling or itching.

If any reaction beyond localized pain, swelling, and itching is experienced, including extensive hives or difficulty breathing, seek prompt medical assistance.

Cone-nose bug, a.k.a. the "kissing bug" (subfamily Triatominae)

The parasitic, blood-sucking cone-nose assassin bug has the potential to be a bigger problem. About an inch long, black, and trimmed with reddish orange marks along its edges, the triatomine is indigenous to both North and South America. Nicknamed the "kissing bug" for its unsavory habit of seeking a blood meal from the soft tissue of the lips and eyes of its sleeping victims, the bug can spread Chagas disease and also cause serious allergic reactions.

Infected triatomines have been found in Florida, along with Chagas-infected populations of raccoons, resulting in Florida Department of Health statements on the potential for the disease here.[5] But so far, there have been no reports of triatomine-induced Chagas in Florida.

More to our purposes, triatomines can cause allergies via the salivary proteins they inject during the process of obtaining their blood meal.[6] Cases of severe allergic reactions to several species of triatomines, including our native *Triatoma sanguisuga*, have been reported throughout the western and southwestern United States, Hawaii, and much of South America.

Cone-nose "kissing bugs," while not a serious issue in Florida at the moment, are considered a species of concern, and Floridians are advised to be aware of some of the characteristics of triatomine bites, which are usually painless due to an anesthetic contained in

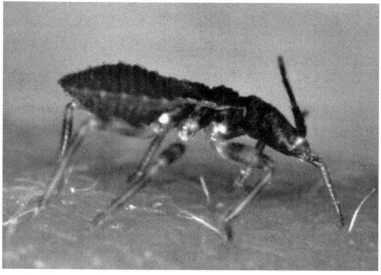

Triatoma infestans or the "kissing bug," "assassin bug," or "cone-nose bug," is a vector for Chagas disease. (Centers for Disease Control and Prevention's Public Health Image Library [PHIL], identification number #2538.)

the bug's saliva. Common reactions to this assassin bug bite can include intense itching of the extremities, redness and swelling, and rapid heartbeat.[7]

The University of Arizona Extension Service observes that cone-nose bug bites have some distinguishing features that can help differentiate them from other insect bites.

- Victims may awaken with unexplained nodules.
- Multiple bites appear in clusters on one part of the body.
- Bites are found on areas of the body not covered by clothing or bedding.
- Lesions are bigger and itchier than those from other insect bites.

In areas where cone-nose bug bites are common, sensitivities can develop after an initial bite. Beyond the usual washing and topical antihistamine lotions or creams, though, no other treatment is usually necessary. Those exhibiting more serious reactions should visit a doctor promptly.

There's usually no reason to control assassin bugs like wheel bugs in Florida, since they're important beneficial insects, and they're simply not that abundant in residential areas.

Triatoma aren't a problem for hikers, although campers should take precautions, especially at night. Secure tent openings, cover well at night (triatoma typically only bite exposed areas) and use insect netting.

To protect against water bugs and other assassin bugs, like wheel bugs, wear proper shoes and clothing when outside. Wear waders or closed-toe shoes when in the water, and gloves, and snug clothing around neck areas when working in gardens or hiking.

Bed bugs (family Cimicidae)—Allergy potential: Moderate

"Sleep tight and don't let the bed bugs bite" was my nightly childhood benediction, as if this would somehow help me sleep better.

I never had a bed bug encounter as a child, but my chances of having one now have greatly improved. Once the scourge of old English inns, bed bugs were, until relatively recently, only rarely encountered and only in less-than-reputable places. But the bed bug is making a comeback, with reports up 71 percent in the United States since 2004.[8] Infestations have become so prevalent that the Environmental Protection Agency has begun hosting annual bed bug summits to examine ways of dealing with the pest.[9]

The 2010 Bed Bug Summit came on the heels of a massive bed bug outbreak that closed stores in New York City in July and August of 2010. "They're like the Taliban hiding in the mountains of Afghanistan," noted one attendee.[10] Indeed, in 2009 alone, NYC recorded more than 11,000 complaints about bed bugs, up from a little over 500 in 2004.[11] The problem has become so intractable that a New York policy group created a website called *New York vs. Bed Bugs* to archive research and news about the issue.

In Florida, the dominant species is *cimix hemipterus*, or the tropical bed bug. As of the summer of 2009, the bed bug registry showed nearly 280 reports of bed bugs in hotels and apartments across the

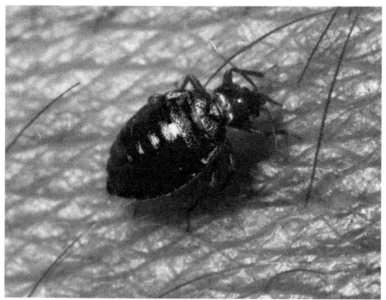

Bed bug. (Photo courtesy of Clemson University, USDA Cooperative Extension Slide Series, Bugwood.org. This work is licensed under a Creative Commons Attribution 3.0 License.)

state; not just in the expected no-star roadside rental of last resort, but in luxury hotels in Orlando, Tampa, and Miami.

Bed bugs are tiny, oval insects, about a quarter of an inch long, and wingless. Most people don't ever feel a bed bug bite. Like triatomines, they feed at night, drawn to the carbon dioxide exhalations of their sleeping victims. Their saliva contains an anticoagulant that expedites their blood meal and also causes varying degrees of itching and swelling in victims, sometimes resulting in severe allergic reactions, and often in considerable psychological distress.[12]

Although bed bugs may host the organisms that cause hepatitis B and Chagas disease, they've never traditionally been considered true carriers of disease. However, a recent Canadian study has found that bed bugs can harbor methicillin-resistant *Staphylococcus aureus* (MRSA) and vancomycin-resistant *Enterococcus faecium* (VRE), two common and potentially deadly forms of drug resistant bacteria. Contaminated bed bugs "may promote the spread of MRSA in impoverished and overcrowded communities," said the researchers, concluding, "Bed bugs carrying MRSA and/or VRE may have the potential to act as vectors for transmission." The report recommends further study.[13]

Most bed bug encounters, however, are more of a nuisance than anything else. Signs of bites are usually small itchy red welts, sometimes in clusters or swaths of three, known as the "breakfast, lunch, and dinner" pattern, indicating repeated feedings by one bed bug.[14] More severe reactions, indicating allergic sensitivity, can include large, itching wheals up to eight inches across, blister-like skin inflammations, and hive-like skin rashes.

In a curious twist of fate, increased exposure to bed bug bites appears to confer some immunity. Although bed bugs can be difficult to control, Florida's bed bugs are comparatively weak next to the "mutant bed bugs" of New York. According to a 2009 *Journal of Medical Entomology* report, New York City bed bugs are now 264 times more resistant to deltamethrin, a common bed bug insecticide, than Florida bed bugs.[15]

Joked one Gotham City blogger, "Of course, Florida is where bed bugs retire to suck blood in their old age, so it figures they'd have a higher mortality rate there."[16]

Maybe so, but even in Florida they can be difficult to detect, and hard to eradicate.

Bed Bug Habitat

Bed bugs can thrive in Florida, especially in crowded, multifamily places like apartments, hotels, cruise ships, hospitals, and dormitories. They can also be transported into homes via luggage and pets. During the day, they hide in cracks and crevices, in wall outlets, along and behind baseboards, and in and around beds, mattresses, and linens, making them difficult to detect.

Signs of severe infestations may include tiny feces on sheets or mattress, quarter-inch-long reddish-brown discs of shed bed bug skins, and a sweet, musty odor.

Bed bugs typically require humans for survival, but they can and will live off rodents and birds. They can also survive for up to six months without a host and have been found to live up to a year in abandoned homes.[17]

Treating Bed Bug Bites

Treat bed bug bites by washing bite sites thoroughly and applying a topical antihistamine or corticosteroid to relieve itching and swelling. Scratching bites can break the skin and cause secondary infections. Oral antihistamines may be prescribed for severe reactions.

Control and Prevention of Bed Bugs

The University of Florida has come up with an innovative treatment for dorm infestations—a portable bed-sized oven that heats mattresses and dressers to 113 degrees.[18] The device has proven effective and eliminated the need for the large-scale fumigation methods used in the past.

In private homes, control is mostly a matter of prevention. Bed bugs won't stay on a host, but if exposure to bed bugs while traveling is suspected, clean everything thoroughly before bringing clothing and luggage indoors. Potentially infested clothing should be washed and dried on hot settings.[19]

Other preventative measures include

- carefully inspecting secondhand furniture before bringing it in;
- changing bed linens weekly and washing them in hot water;
- vacuuming weekly, especially around baseboards, beds, and furniture posts; and
- caulking and chemically treating any cracks or crevices in the home.

Infestation control measures include extensive dusting and spraying of appropriate pesticides in all crevices and cracks, drawers, box springs, baseboards, and carpeting, as well as vacuuming thoroughly and disposing of the vacuum cleaner bag or contents in a sealed plastic bag.

Lice (order Phthiraptera)—Allergy potential: Significant

Lice are tiny, a couple of millimeters at most, and virtually identical the world over, with minor adaptations for ethnic populations.[20] There are three types of human lice—body, head, and pubic. Body and pubic lice infestations (crabs) result from poor hygiene and sexual contact and are not discussed here.

Head lice infestations (pediculosis), however, are common in schools and daycare centers throughout the United States, with an estimated 6 to 12 million infestations annually nationwide among children aged 3 to 11. Cleanliness or a lack thereof is not a factor in the spread of head lice, which travels via head-to-head contact and, less commonly, via shared clothing, hair care items, towels, and linens.

While head lice aren't implicated in the spread of disease, and victims are often actually asymptomatic during initial or light infestations, allergic pruritus, or severe itching, can occur and may produce secondary infections as a result of excessive scratching. Symptoms can take up to six weeks to appear after an initial infestation and may include (as will probably occur while you read this) a tickling sensation or a feeling of something moving in the hair, irritability and sleeplessness, and sores resulting from scratching.

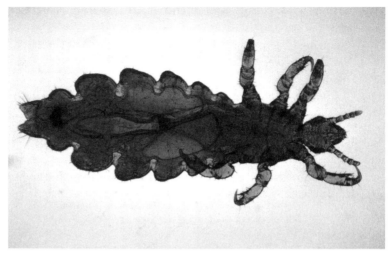

Dorsal view of a female head louse, *Pediculus humanus var. capitis*. (Photo by Dr. Dennis D. Juranek, CDC.)

Treating Head Lice Infestations

Head lice infestations are treated with over-the-counter or prescription scalp medications, removal of nits (eggs), thorough household cleaning, and retreatment in nine or ten days. Head lice can't survive without their human host for more than two days, nor can nits hatch, so removing all possibility of reinfection is the goal of treatment.

Furniture and floors must be vacuumed thoroughly to remove any infested hairs that might have been shed. Combs and brushes must be soaked in hot water, and everything used or worn by the infected person just prior to treatment should be laundered and dried on the hottest settings, dry-cleaned, or sealed in plastic bags for two weeks.

Lice Control

The best way to control lice is to prevent them in the first place. The chances of head lice infestation can be greatly reduced by educating children about healthy play and socializing, and ensuring that schools and daycare centers have healthy policies in place. To preventing head lice infestations,

- discourage head-to-head or hair-to-hair contact during play and activities, including sports, slumber parties, and camping;
- discourage sharing of clothing, stuffed toys, and personal hair care items;
- avoid reclining on beds, pillows, or carpets that may have been in contact with an infested person; and
- follow head lice treatment procedures completely to avoid recurrence and further spread of lice.

Fleas (order Siphonaptera)—Allergy potential: Slight

Dog owners in Florida probably wouldn't be surprised to learn that their dogs have fleas. However, it might be surprising to learn they are probably cat fleas. In fact, the cat flea (*Ctenocephalides felis felis*) is the most common domestic flea and the flea most often found in Florida. The dog flea is rare in the United States, occurring generally in Europe.[21]

Although there are thousands of flea species, usually adapted to live on a particular host, most people will only encounter the cat flea and possibly the sticktight flea, a poultry specialist that will occasionally hitch a ride and feed on other domestic animals.

Fleas are tiny creatures with an oversized jump—some can spring up to 13 inches, over 200 times their own body length—and they have an equally oversized bite applied as readily to humans as to a specific animal host.

Historically, fleas have been responsible for the spread of flea-borne typhus and the plague—it wasn't the rats but their fleas.[22] Even today, the World Health Organization reports 1,000 to 3,000 cases of plague annually worldwide.

On animals, fleas can cause physical distress, hair loss, tapeworms, and other infections. Serious and uncontrolled pet infestations, or even the absence of a pet for a while (and therefore the usual meal), can leave hapless humans covered in irritating, itchy papules, often in that "breakfast, lunch, and dinner" pattern that suggests one has become a human buffet. Pets often develop allergic reactions to fleas; humans not so often. But bites can become swollen, inflamed, and infected from excessive scratching, and on rare occasions, more serious allergic responses can develop.

Bites often occur around bends and folds in the skin, around the waist, ankles, armpits, and behind and inside of knees, and elbows.[23] Within hours of flea bites, human victims can develop hives, localized or generalized itching, and sometimes swelling around an existing sore or injury.

Flea Habitat

Fleas are superbly adapted parasites, not only latterly flattened to better pass through forests of hair, but with barbed feet and anteriorially pointing bristles that complicate flea removal. Animals have their own adaptations to cope with their fleas; cats' sandpapery tongues effectively help comb fleas from their fur, for instance.

Treating Flea Bites

Bites can usually be easily treated with hydrocortisone or other over-the-counter anti-itch, antihistamine creams and medications.

Controlling Fleas

The best way to discourage fleas is to make their preferred habitat—pets and yards—uninviting. Typically, if fleas are controlled on pets, they won't pose a problem elsewhere. So protected pets are the best line of defense, and prescription spot-on tick and flea treatments are the gold standard. While flea collars, store-brand treatments, and home foggers are less expensive, they're also less reliable and sometimes dangerous to use. Coordinating treatment with a veterinarian is the most effective way to keep pets healthy and homes flea-free.

Yard treatments can also help. Flea larvae prefer shade and humidity, but avoid flooded areas. A good rainfall or even a good spray with a hose often curbs flea development outdoors. Outdoor insecticide sprays and treatments applied during the dry season help protect against fleas during more hospitable flea weather. Biological controls with beneficial nematodes have also proven effective.[24]

Biting Flies (order Diptera)

Next to Hymenoptera, insects of the order Diptera, or true flies, cause the most problems. These include the blood-feeding deer and horse flies, mosquitoes, and biting midges. They are also vectors of some of the most serious diseases on our planet and are potentially allergenic.

Fly bites can cause both localized and generalized IgE-mediated allergic reactions, usually to the anticoagulant enzymatic proteins in fly saliva that expedite their blood meal. Both mosquitoes and horse flies have been known to cause anaphylactic shock in highly sensitive individuals.[25]

Horse and Deer Flies (family Tabanidae)—Allergy potential: Moderate to High

There are about 100 species of horse and deer flies in Florida, thanks in great measure to our abundance of water, which flies require for breeding. The behavior and life cycles of horse flies—a jet black fly with huge eyes—and deer flies—which are smaller and honey colored (hence their other name, "yellow flies")—are similar. Only the female of each species bites, while the males of each species are nectar feeders.[26] Allergic reactions to bites of both of these flies can cause significant urticaria and occasionally anaphylaxis.[27]

Horse fly bites are especially painful due to their nightmarish beak of a mouth, which literally saws its way through the flesh of man or beast. Horse flies usually bite along the victim's head, neck, or upper torso. Deer flies generally strike around the arms and lower extremities and can be relentless assailants during their peak seasons in late spring and early fall.[28] The deer fly will also bite when trapped indoors, unlike most other flies of this family.[29]

Tabanid Habitat

Horse and deer flies are mostly sight hunters, attracted to dark colors and motion, but they are also drawn to scents and the carbon dioxide exhalations of potential prey. They usually shelter in shady places in brush and under trees. Horse flies are most active before noon and

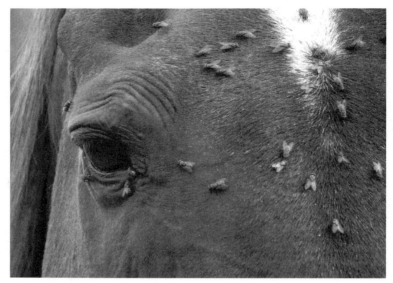

Horse flies on horse. (Photo by Jina Lee, ©2007. Permission is granted to copy, distribute, and/or modify this document under the terms of the GNU Free Documentation License, version 1.2 or any later version published by the Free Software Foundation.)

just prior to and through sunset. They're often inactive during very cool, very hot, or overcast weather.[30]

Deer flies, on the other hand, will attack throughout the day, most heavily in the late afternoon. They tend to be more active on cloudy days, especially near water, although they rarely stray far from the cover of trees.[31] While it might be easy to hear, or at least see, a big black horse fly lumbering nearby, deer flies are the stealth bombers of the fly world, appearing out of nowhere to stab a leg or arm.

Treating Tabanid Bites

Tabanid bites are usually painful. Promptly applying an ammonia-based bite neutralizer may alleviate symptoms. Otherwise, topical anesthetics containing benzocaine or lidocaine may help. Over-the-counter antihistamine creams or oral medications can help reduce swelling and itching, as can hydrocortisone creams.

Controlling Tabanids

Biting flies can be difficult to control, although there are some reliable standards.

- Biological controls like cattle egrets, killdeer, and some varieties of wasps will control biting fly populations.
- Pruning or removing underbrush and weedy areas can reduce biting flies by removing shelter and increasing air flow.
- Using fans on porches, patios, and picnic areas will discourage flies, which prefer still air.
- Burning citronella candles, coils, and torches can help.
- Chemical controls can be applied in cracks and crevices and around window frames and doors if flies are appearing indoors.
- A wide range of traps—malaise traps that lure flies with CO_2, octenol attractants, wind motion traps, and trolling traps—can help reduce populations in small areas.
- County mosquito control services may have a biting fly management program.[32]

Outdoor Protection against Biting Flies

Avoiding the outdoors during periods of tabanid activity is the most effective way to protect against bites. Biting flies are usually active early in the day and in the afternoon, especially near water, and usually in greatest abundance in the fall. Deer flies are most active in May and June. Undeterred outdoors lovers can take other precautions.

- Wear long-sleeved shirts and long pants.
- Use insect repellent: repellents containing DEET are the most effective on skin; permethrin is used on clothing.
- Try a trolling deer fly trap!

The trolling deer fly trap was developed by the University of Florida's North Florida Entomology Research and Education Center.[33] The homemade contraption catches both deer flies and horse flies in a rather eye-catching and, to read the accolades about the trap, often entertaining manner.

Traps can be made from buckets, flower pots, cups, and even hats that are painted a bright blue (one satisfied reviewer reported great success with Rustoleum number 7724 "sail blue") and coated with Tanglefoot, a sticky insect trap coating available at garden supply stores.

Alone and unmoving, the trap doesn't do much. But placed on a slow-moving vehicle, mounted on a stick or pole, and shaken over a walker's head or worn atop the head (preferably in the form of a cup or hat, rather than a flower pot or bucket!), the trolling fly trap appears remarkably effective. One user reported capturing 150 flies on a Tanglefoot-coated blue beach pail. Others reported that a few forays with a trolling trap reduced fly populations to tolerable levels for outdoor work.

So for those willing to wear sticky hats, the trolling fly trap might just be the ticket for controlling tabanids outdoors!

Stable Flies (*Stomoxys calcitrans*)—Allergy potential: Slight

Similar to a house fly in appearance, the stable fly, also known as the dog fly, is a common, exasperating and costly pest throughout Florida, especially in West Florida along the Gulf Coast, where it can be a bane to beachgoers. The fly breeds in stable debris, hence its name, as well as among decaying seaweed along beaches.

The flies regularly shelter on leeward sides of dunes, where they become persistent and painful pests, resisting all attempts at dissuasion and, at certain times of the year, often resulting in a shortened day at the beach. They can also take up residence on boats and wreak havoc on an afternoon on the water. Both genders of this species bite. They are most common in the morning, and a change of wind as the day progresses can sweep the flies away with welcome suddenness.[34]

Mosquitoes (family Culicidae)—Allergy potential: Moderate to High

The mosquito is an ancient fly, virtually unchanged over 30 million years, and one of the most dangerous insects in the world, spreading everything from malaria to several different types of encephalitis, including West Nile virus, which occurs in Florida. There are about 80 species of mosquitoes in Florida. As with many other fly species, only the female bites; males, distinguished by their feathery antennae, feed on nectar.

Almost anyone who sets foot in Florida will have an encounter with mosquitoes. Most victims develop the characteristic little itchy red bump that lasts a day or two and often experience lessening reactions throughout mosquito season. A small number of people, however, will experience a more widespread IgE antibody response to the proteins in mosquito saliva and develop larger swellings, sometimes skin blisters, and suffer bruising or hives that may last one or more weeks. More rarely, anaphylaxis may occur.[35]

Mosquitoes, as any outdoors person knows, have unerring aim when it comes to homing in on any exposed patch of skin, and they can even attack through clothing. Mosquitoes find blood meals in several ways. They use chemical sensors that can detect carbon dioxide and lactic acid from as far as 100 feet away, visual cues triggered by motion and contrasting colors, and heat detectors that lure them to warm-blooded animals.[36]

Mosquitoes are most active at dawn and dusk, especially in moist, shady, and wind-protected areas. With each mosquito bite, it's safe to assume the mosquito has either just laid eggs—to the tune of about 200–300 at a time—or is just about to, since the protein from a blood meal is required for egg development.

Our slap and scratch response to mosquito bites is the result of their injection of anticoagulants into our skin. These proteins prevent clotting and enable a freer flow from the blood tap at the shin bar. *Aedes aegypti*, a common Florida mosquito, can tip back about five microliters per serving.

For most of us, the itching persists until immune cells successfully break down the irritating saliva proteins. For a small handful of folks, their immune system can't cope, and the swelling and itching may extend far beyond the site of mosquito bites.

Mosquito Myths

Since the mosquito is such a ubiquitous part of Florida life, a variety of tales have sprung up around the insect.

Myth: Mosquitoes in Florida can be two inches long.

Fact: No, they can't. They just feel that big when they bite. In fact,

Florida's (and the nation's) largest mosquito, *Psorophora ciliata*, is less than a half inch long. What many report as huge mosquitoes are actually nectar-feeding crane flies, large, bumbling, dangly legged insects that closely resemble mosquitoes but have none of their bad habits.

Myth: Mosquitoes transmit AIDS.

Fact: They can transmit a lot of things, but not AIDS, and for a couple of reasons:

1. The AIDS virus is digested by the mosquito and can't be transmitted intact.
2. While the bite may feel needlelike, the mosquito's proboscis does not function as a hypodermic needle, but like a unidirectional valve allowing blood to flow into the mosquito, not out. The salivary proteins that trigger itching and allergies are delivered via another mouthpart, not the proboscis.[37]

Myth: Ultrasonic devices will repel mosquitoes.

Fact: No, they won't, nor will bug zappers, or even birds or bats, which just don't eat enough of the insects to make a significant difference. The best way to reduce mosquitoes around a home is to keep areas free of standing water that supports breeding.[38]

Mosquito Habitat

Mosquitoes and water go together like, well—mosquitoes and water. Generally, all mosquitoes require standing water or moist soil to breed, although different species prefer different types of water environments, ranging from fresh to salt, and from moldering organic material, to contained water in things like tires or buckets, to swamps and marshes.[39]

Eggs hatch into larvae known as "wigglers," which often serve as tasty snacks for fish and other predators and also as a wakeup call when found in a neglected birdbath.

Treating Mosquito Bites

Wash mosquito bites with soap and water, and use over-the-counter antihistamines creams or lotions or calamine lotion to relieve itching. Avoid scratching bites to prevent secondary infections. If dizziness, nausea, or extensive itching and swelling are experienced, seek prompt medical attention as these may indicate a severe allergic reaction. People with known mosquito allergies should avoid mosquito-infested areas and periods of high mosquito activity during mornings, late afternoons and early evening.

Mosquito Control

Mosquito control is usually undertaken on a large scale throughout Florida, with neighborhood fogging trucks making the rounds seasonally when mosquitoes are breeding and active. Residents experiencing severe mosquito problems in their communities should check with the local mosquito control agency for county or city control programs.

Around a home, mosquito problems can be significantly alleviated by

- eliminating areas of debris and standing water;
- flushing birdbaths and decorative fountains with fresh water regularly to discourage wigglers;
- keeping window and door screens in good condition; and
- stocking ornamental ponds and fountains with mosquito-eating fish.

Outdoor Protection against Mosquitoes

The best way to protect against mosquitoes is to avoid them—a tricky proposition in Florida. Who wants to miss out on boating, fishing, hiking, wildlife, bird-watching, and even hanging out at the beach because of mosquitoes? If we stop enjoying our great outdoors, the bugs win! But a little outdoor savvy can be helpful.

- Avoid mosquito habitat—persistently wet or damp, shady, or swampy areas, especially during rainy seasons, at dawn or dusk, or on windless days.
- Wear appropriate clothing during mosquito season (basically warm rainy weather): lightweight, light-colored, long-sleeved shirts and pants. Loose-fitting clothing makes it harder for mosquitoes to bite, but also easier for some other insects to get inside clothing.

- Apply mosquito repellent to skin and clothing. Repellents containing DEET are considered the most effective, but the Centers for Disease Control and Prevention also found repellents containing picaridin and oil of lemon eucalyptus to be effective.

The Dope on DEET

DEET has been mentioned a few times in this chapter and will be mentioned again. DEET is shorthand for N,N-Diethyl-meta-toluamide, a chemical insect repellent developed by the U.S. Army in 1946 for soldiers engaged in jungle warfare. It was registered for commercial use in 1956 and remains the most effective insect repellent for discouraging biting flies, midges, mosquitoes, and ticks.[40]

It is also considered a Category III "slightly toxic" chemical by the Environmental Protection Agency (EPA). DEET is a known eye and, sometimes, skin irritant that has been implicated in seizures in children. Public debates about its safety have confused and concerned people for years. However, concerns about the possible effects of occasional use have to be weighed against the potential for injury and sickness that can result from insect bites and stings.

In reregistering DEET for public use in 1998, the EPA took into consideration reports of seizures attributed to DEET and concluded, "Given only 14 to 32 cases since 1960 (the first case was reported in 1961) and 50–80 million people using DEET each year, the observed incidence of recognized seizures is about one per 100 million users."[41]

Insect repellents are marketed with varying amounts of DEET, the most expensive containing the highest concentration of the repellent. There's a tipping point for DEET's effectiveness, though. Army studies found that concentrations of 30–40 percent DEET worked twice as well as concentrations of 75 percent.[42] Anything containing between 20 and 40 percent DEET will be sufficient in protecting against mosquitoes for a reasonable amount of time.

Apply according to directions and use carefully around the face. Picaridin and eucalyptus oil show promise as DEET alternatives and, unlike DEET, they don't dissolve plastics.

Biting Midges (family Ceratopogonidae)—Allergy potential: Moderate

Also known as sandflies, no-see-ums, or punkies, biting midges are infinitesimal flies with disproportionately big bites. It's probably the smallest biting insect you'll never see, easily mistaken for a speck of dirt. But it's not hard to imagine that the insect is all mouth—a sharp, pointy, painful little stabbing mouth.

There are nearly 50 species of biting midges in Florida, although only about half a dozen pester people, mostly in coastal areas. Between an eighth and a sixteenth of an inch in size, they easily squeeze through screens. As with many other biting flies, only the female midge feeds on blood, breaking through capillaries in the skin, minutely but often painfully, via small cutting teeth on its elongated mandibles. Like the other biting flies, it injects an anticoagulant into

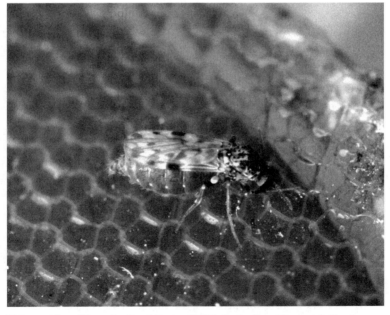

Biting midge. (Photo by Scott Bauer, USDA Agricultural Research Service, Bugwood.org. Creative Commons Attribution 3.0 License.)

the wound to expedite feeding. Some people are sensitive to the proteins in the midges' saliva and can experience generalized allergic reactions.

Horses, oddly enough, are often hypersensitive to biting midges and can develop an allergic dermatitis response known as "sweet itch," which plagues stables nationwide. The midge species, *C. furens* and *C. barbosai*, can also spread *Mansonella ozzardi*, a human nematode parasite that causes skin lesions and dermatitis. Fortunately, the disease does not seem to be endemic in Florida.[43]

Biting Midge Habitat

Biting midges are mostly a summer problem, although depending on weather and location, they may bite throughout the year in Florida. Midges are common in swampy areas and intertidal zones, especially at low tide. Most no-see-ums breed in salt marshes, but some breed in freshwater environments as well, amounting to a breeding area that's basically all of Florida.[44]

A good stiff breeze may whisk them away, but they're quick to return and almost impossible to deter. They're especially attracted to high body temperatures and perspiration, annoying more vigorously the harder one labors.

Biting Midge Control

Control of biting midges is almost impossible. They live everywhere and may seem to emerge continually. Some believe climate change might be responsible for increases in biting midge populations, which thrive in warm water environments that promote the growth of the algae and phytoplankton on which larvae feed.[45]

"Impounding"—flooding swampy areas—has proven helpful in some areas by disrupting midge breeding and egg-laying habitats, although this can be environmentally counterproductive.[46] CO_2 traps, used mostly on islands, can also help.[47] But midges remain persistent throughout much of Florida.

At a residential level, utilizing small-mesh screens and keeping them in good repair can help keep no-see-ums out of homes and patios. Screens can also be treated with insect repellents. Ceiling and window fans set on high also discourage the insects, which are easily blown away because of their minute size and poor flying ability.[48]

Outdoor Protection against Midges

Most of the guidance for protecting against mosquitoes applies to biting midges. Dress appropriately, avoid outdoor activity during periods of midge activity—hot, still weather near the water—and apply appropriate insect repellents to skin and clothing.

Nonbiting Midges (family Chironomidae)—Allergy Potential: High

In one of those darned if they do and darned if they don't twists of fate, the non-biting midges, collectively known as chironomids, possess an allergy potential as great as that of cockroaches and dust mites.[49]

Considered a beneficial insect—and great bait!—in its larval stage, and an indicator of water quality, non-biting midges occur in vast numbers in and around all bodies of water, natural and man-made, inland and coastal. They're an important part of the food chain, providing food for a variety of insect eaters from dragonflies to fish.

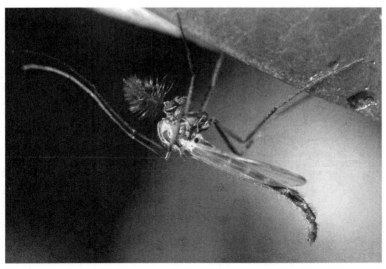

Nonbiting midge. (©Entomart.ins Creative Commons Attribution 3.0 License.)

They're similar in appearance to mosquitoes, right down to the hair-raising whine of their collective and characteristically bumbling flight, hence the nickname "blind mosquitoes."[50] But they don't bite, and they don't even feed for the short one or two days they're alive for the sole purpose of breeding, which they do with great vigor. Their larvae, commonly known as blood worms and prized among fishermen and hobby aquarists, can occur in such abundance, especially in nutrient-rich waters, that densities of over 4,000 larvae per two feet are not unusual. The resulting emergence of all those midges three days later can produce swarms of alarming proportions. Emerging midges are drawn to porch lights and street lights, and in some communities, especially around lakefront homes, piles of midge corpses can cover patios, driveways, and streets, even staining walls and cars with droppings and other secretions.[51]

The midge swarms also stimulate opportunistic spiders to build webs in equal abundance, creating a secondary problem for the arachnophobic. Midge swarms can clog home air conditioners and car radiators, and accumulations of dead midges can become malodorous and even create hazardous street conditions.

These mass emergences are not new in Florida. While cruising the St. Johns River in 1831, John James Audubon reported that midges were so abundant they covered the boat and even extinguished candle flames in cabins. Similar stories from the turn of the twentieth century report swarms of nonbiting midges so large they could put out bonfires and signal lights.

They also cause allergies at surprisingly high rates. It turns out that about 20 percent of people exposed to midges and their larvae develop inhalation allergies, principally bronchial asthma and rhinitis, as well as conjunctivitis.[52]

Studies identify the primary allergic trigger as chironomid hemoglobin,[53] the protein molecule in red blood cells, which gives blood worms their bright red color and their name and which adult midges also possess in great measure. The rich hemoglobin composition allows the larvae to breath in the low-dissolved-oxygen conditions of the lake bottom muck that is their home.[54]

Research has also identified a link between cockroach allergenicity and that of chironomids, as well as a relationship between mosquito allergy and chironomid allergy and between dust mite allergy and chironimid allergy. Further, chironomid-specific IgE antibodies show up in individuals who have never even been exposed to midges.[55]

Those at risk include people living near chironomid breeding areas and those who work with blood worms and fish food occupationally or recreationally, like the hobby aquarist.[56]

Chironomid Habitat

Chironomids need water to breed, since larvae filter feed on algae and lake detritus in muddy lakes and ponds of all sizes, as well as in slow-moving shallow creeks and rivers. Chironomid life spans cycle rapidly every three weeks during the summer and suspend development during the winter, emerging again in the spring.[57] In some places in Florida, emergence can occur throughout the year.

Treating Chironomid Allergy

Individuals experiencing rhinitis, conjunctivitis, and bronchial symptoms every time nonbiting midges swarm can probably assume an allergy to chironomids. Minor symptoms can be alleviated by simply staying indoors when midges are active or wearing a dust or particle mask when outdoors during emergence periods. Over-the-counter antihistamines may also help.[58] If the problem is severe, an allergist should be consulted.

Chironomid Control

Individuals and communities can take several steps to prevent overpopulations of nonbiting midges, while also improving the health of lakes and ponds.

- Limit fertilization of lawns, gardens, golf courses, and fields to reduce the nutrient-rich runoff that leads to the excessive algae growth on which blood worms feed.
- Keep porch lights and flood lights off and window blinds closed to help discourage midges.
- Communities can use specially placed high-intensity white

lights, which help draw midges away from residential areas, or high-pressure sodium lamps, which are less attractive to them.

- Fish and midge-eating insects are good biological controls, so encouraging biodiversity around a healthy pond or lake can help reduce midge populations. A biological larvicide, *Bacillus thuringiensis* var. *israelensis* (Bti), is also effective.

Chemical insecticides, specifically larvicides, can be used as a last resort to control midge larvae in standing water, although these may harm other creatures, like fish, that eat larvae.

Blister Beetles (family Meloidae) and False Blister Beetles (family Oedemeridae)—Allergy potential: Minimal, but can produce contact dermatitis

There are nearly 30 species of blister beetles and false blister beetles in Florida. The two insects are similar in appearance. However, false blister beetles lack a "neck" and are pollen feeders. Blister beetles are herbivorous, dining mostly on flowers but also on some plant leaves, depending on species.[59]

In and of themselves, neither blister nor false blister beetles are a problem. They don't sting or bite. They don't buzz picnickers or beachgoers or insistently pester gardeners or hikers. Some are occasionally beneficial; the larvae of the striped blister beetle feeds on grasshopper eggs, although the adult is considered a crop pest.[60]

However, the blood of both families contains cantharidin, a vesicating, or blistering, agent that can cause painful dermatitis on humans and poisoning in animals like horses that may ingest the dead beetles via hay or other feed. Cantharidin is released from the insects only when they're crushed or pinched, as in reflexive swatting or other accidental contact.[61]

Under ordinary circumstances, cantharidin acts as a predatory defense for the beetles. On people, though, it produces blister beetle dermatitis. Skin blistering begins within 24 hours of contact, after which the blisters can progress to itching and oozing lesions that can become infected. Cantharidin content varies by species, ranging from 1 to 5 percent—minute amounts but sufficiently toxic enough to produce blistering in nearly anyone who encounters blister beetle fluids.[62]

Blister and False Blister Beetle Habitat

The beetles are largely vegetarians, living in agricultural or horticultural areas, and feeding on flowers or leaves. But they are drawn to lights at night, especially in the spring and summer. False blister beetles are especially abundant in the Florida Keys, where they swarm around lights by swimming pools, tennis courts, and outdoor dining areas.[63] Blisters typically result from the insects being squashed, slapped, or brushed away when they alight on necks and arms. Light handling doesn't usually pose a problem, and some people are more susceptible to blistering than others.[64]

Treating Blister Beetle Injuries

Unless blistering is extensive, basic first aid treatment for blisters is usually the most effective treatment. See a doctor for severe blistering and any sign of infection.

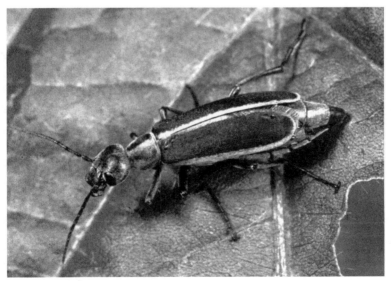

Margined blister beetle. (Photo courtesy of Clemson University—USDA Cooperative Extension Slide Series, Bugwood.org. Creative Commons Attribution 3.0 License.)

Blister Beetle Control

Blister beetles and false blister beetles are best controlled through spot treatment with appropriate pesticides on clearly infected areas of foliage. Since the striped blister beetle larvae feed on grasshopper eggs, reducing grasshopper populations will also reduce striped blister beetle populations.[65]

Outdoor Protection against Blister Beetles

Blister beetles are most active during spring and summer months, usually when residents and visitors are enjoying poolside fun in the evenings or open air dining. Keeping lights away from where people congregate can help keep the beetles away, too. Electronic bug killers also help.

Caterpillars (order Lepidoptera)—Allergy Potential: High

Almost every American child is familiar with Eric Carle's *Very Hungry Caterpillar*. It is the beautiful and richly visual story of a fat, voracious, but good-natured roly-poly caterpillar that eats its way through a veritable orchard of fruits and vegetables and a forest of leaves.

Gardeners may cringe at the very thought. But there's no denying that behind every larval caterpillar is the inspiring transformation of a butterfly or the sometimes darker manifestation of a moth. While caterpillars can, in fact, wreak havoc on a beloved home garden or the life work of a farm, for the most part they don't pose any physical threat to people—except for a small and potent handful.

Injuries usually result from passive, inadvertent encounters with the caterpillars' venomous spines. The venom is thought to contain peptides and histamine-releasing substances that produce rhinitis or dermatitis of varying degrees.

Caterpillars can cause three principal reactions in people:

1. Caterpillar dermatitis (erucism), produced by contact with toxic caterpillar hairs, spines, or fluids in the air or on the caterpillar
2. Lepidopterism, a systemic illness characterized by general

urticaria, respiratory problems, nausea, vomiting, and headaches
3. Opthalmia nodosa—basically acute conjunctivitis caused by
venomous caterpillar hairs in the eyes

In sensitive individuals, IgE antibodies to the venom of an initial
contact result in widespread urticaria or other symptoms upon a
subsequent contact. Even caterpillars without venomous spines can
sometimes produce contact dermatitis in some people. Other people
suffer respiratory allergies from inhaling caterpillar spines.[66]

Florida's "Big Four" caterpillars are all larvae of moths: puss, saddleback, io, and hag. To a lesser degree, the buck moth and spiney
oak slug caterpillars can also trigger allergic symptoms.

Caterpillar Habitat

Flannel moth caterpillars, especially the remarkable puss caterpillars, are considered among the most dangerous in the United States.
They're most active in the spring and fall on oak and citrus trees,
but they feed on a variety of broad-leafed trees and shrubs. As their
names suggests, the puss caterpillar and the adult flannel moth are
furry in appearance.

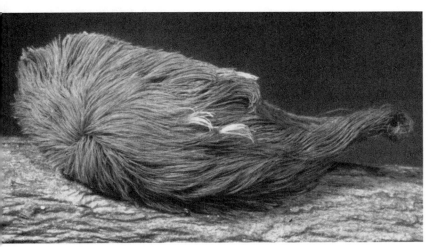

Puss caterpillar. (Photo by Gerald J. Lenhard, Louisiana State University,
Bugwood.org. Creative Commons Attribution 3.0 License.)

While it may appear soft and alluring, particularly to children, the puss caterpillar's looks are definitely deceiving. Beneath the luxuriant coat is an undershirt of stiff, venomous spines that break off in the skin on contact and can cause severe pain.[67] Those with a history of hay fever or asthma are particularly at risk for an allergic reaction.

The saddleback caterpillar is identified by an obvious bright green "saddle" studded with venomous spines fore and aft and around the sides. This is a ubiquitous caterpillar that doesn't seem to show any dining preferences. Contact with the spines can cause severe pain for some people and only minor itching or burning for others.[68]

The io moth is a huge, beautiful moth sporting a pair of blue and yellow eyespots on wings that can measure up to three and a half inches across. Its larvae are pretty, spiky green things with a couple of lateral stripes, the topmost red and the lower one white, that can deliver a painful sting on contact. The caterpillars favor ixora and roses, but can also be found on other plants.

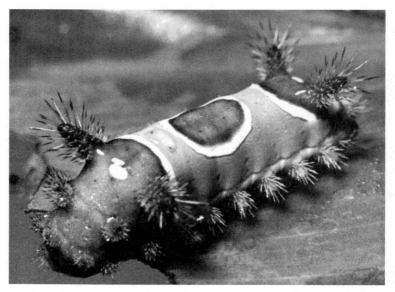

Saddleback caterpillar. (Photo courtesy of Clemson University—USDA Cooperative Extension Slide Series, Bugwood.org. Creative Commons Attribution 3.0 License.)

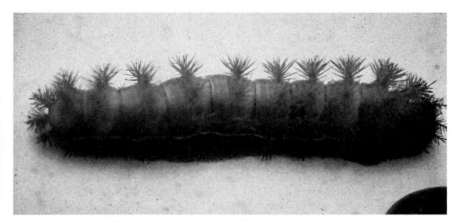

Io moth caterpillar. (Photo courtesy of Center for Disease Control Archive, Centers for Disease Control and Prevention, Bugwood.org. Creative Commons Attribution 3.0 License.)

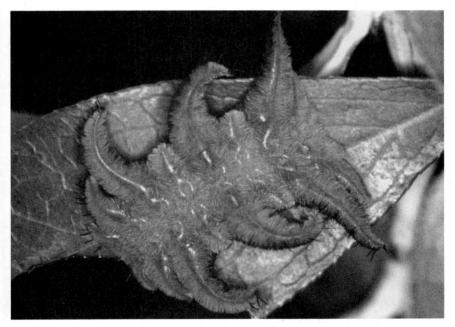

Hag moth caterpillar. (Photo by Jerry A. Payne, USDA Agricultural Research Service, Bugwood.org. Creative Commons Attribution 3.0 License.)

Not quite as common as the others, the hag caterpillar, and its grownup self, the hag moth, can be unsettling looking things, all furry protuberances. Sometimes known as the monkey slug, it feeds on a variety of forest trees and some ornamental shrubs. It has a motley collection of venomous spines that can produce pain and itching on contact.

Treating Caterpillar Stings

Caterpillar hairs adhering to the skin can usually be removed by repeated applications of sticky tape. The site of injury should be washed thoroughly with soap and water and, rather than rubbed dry with a towel, air dried or dried with a hot-air hair dryer. Other helpful measures include

- applying cooling compresses or applications, like topical isopropyl alcohol, ammonia, or ice packs;
- flushing eyes with water in the event of ophthalmic contact;
- using over-the-counter antihistamines or topical corticosteroids to relieve itching and swelling; and
- elevating the injured area.

If serious allergic symptoms develop, especially respiratory problems, seek immediate medical care.

Caterpillar Control

Most caterpillar encounters are occasional and accidental, so control may be unnecessary. But for overly abundant caterpillar populations, biological controls like the *Bacillus thuringiensis kurstaki* pathogen can be effective.[69]

Outdoor Protection against Caterpillars

The easiest way to protect against stinging caterpillars is to wear appropriate clothing like gloves and long sleeves when gardening or working outdoors. When hiking, avoid grabbing onto branches or bushes or reaching into hidden areas. And discourage children from playing with hairy caterpillars!

In Summary

- Of the true bugs, assassin bugs pose the biggest threat, especially the so-called "kissing bug" that can spread Chagas disease and cause allergic reactions. While there are no reported cases of Chagas in Florida, infected triatomines have been found here, and the Florida Department of Health recommends ongoing awareness.
- Bed bugs can cause severe dermatological and respiratory allergies in sensitive individuals and pose an increasing problem nationwide. Severe reactions to bites can include blisters and hives. To prevent home infestations, travel items should be cleaned before being brought inside, and clothing and linens should be washed and dried on hot settings.
- Of the three types of lice that afflict humans, human head lice are the most common. They typically affect school children and their families and occasionally may cause allergic pruritis and secondary infections from excessive scratching. Children should be counseled to avoid head-to-head play and to avoid sharing hair care items or hats. Infestations are treated with over-the-counter or prescription medications, by thoroughly cleaning linens and other textiles, and by extensive vacuuming.
- The cat flea is the most common flea in Florida. It affects cats and dogs equally and irritates humans, who can be bitten in the absence of pets or as the result of severe flea infestations in and around homes. Fleas cause more psychological distress than physical injury in humans, although they can cause allergies in hypersensitive individuals. Flea bites are best treated with over-the-counter antihistamine creams. Routinely treating pets with anti-flea medications discourages flea infestations.
- Biting flies (tabanids), namely horse and deer flies, are frequent pests of humans and animals. Tabanid bites are painful and can produce allergic reactions in sensitive individuals. Protect against tabanids by (1) using approved insect repel-

lents, (2) dressing appropriately for the outdoors, (3) reducing tabanid habitat, and (4) avoiding areas where they're active, especially in the morning and late afternoon. Bites are treated with topical anesthetics and hydrocortisone creams.

- A common complaint among Floridians, mosquito bites can sometimes produce severe allergic reactions in sensitive individuals. The best remedy is mosquito control, which mainly involves reducing mosquito habitat (eliminating standing water around the house, for example) and taking simple precautionary measures outdoors, such as wearing appropriate clothing and using insect repellent. In recommended concentrations of 30–40 percent, DEET remains the most effective repellent. Mosquito bites can be treated with ammonia-based itch neutralizers and topical or oral antihistamines.

- Biting midges (no-see-ums) are minute creatures with a painful bite to which some people develop allergies. Avoiding the outdoors during periods of high midge activity (still, hot days) and wearing appropriate insect repellent are the most effective ways to protect against them.

- Non-biting midges, or chironomids, swarm in huge numbers almost year-round in some parts of Florida, especially in the summer, and can cause respiratory allergies in people sensitive to chironomid hemoglobin. Hypersensitive individuals can develop bronchial asthma, rhinitis, and conjunctivitis. Treatment of chironomid allergy involves staying indoors when midges swarm, wearing a dust mask outside, and taking antihistamines. Maintaining healthy ecosystems free of excess nutrients, installing appropriate lighting, and utilizing biological controls can also reduce chironomid populations.

- Blister beetles and false blister beetles can produce severe contact dermatitis when crushed or pinched because of cantharidin, a blistering toxin in their blood. Skin injury can usually be treated with standard first aid for blisters.

- Of the myriad caterpillars in Florida, four cause the greatest number of allergic reactions in humans: the puss, io, hag, and saddleback moth caterpillars. All have venom-charged spines that can cause dermatitis, lepidopterism, and acute conjunctivitis. Chances of injury can be reduced by wearing gloves and appropriate clothing when working outdoors. Treatment of stings includes removing caterpillar hairs from the skin with adhesive tape, washing and air drying the sting site, flushing the eyes thoroughly with water in the case of ophthalmic injury, applying cooling compresses, using over-the-counter antihistamines or analgesics, and elevating the injured area. Consult a doctor for severe reactions.

Part III

Allergies in the Garden of Eden

Many things grow in the garden that were never sown there.

Thomas Fuller, *Gnomologia*, 1732

Florida historians are fond of romanticizing Spanish explorer Juan Ponce de León's discovery of our state. He did, in fact, lead the first European expedition here, looking for the reputed Fountain of Youth and evidence supporting legends of abundant gold and silver. Not fast up on his geology, he came confidently ashore in March 1513 near present-day St. Augustine and proudly planted the Spanish flag. Oblivious to the fact that sedimentary rock isn't a hotbed for precious metals, or that our waters teemed only with fish, alligators, and mosquitoes, he christened the place La Florida, the "place of flowers," and set about trying to get rich quick.

Eight years later, Florida killed him—or, more precisely, a Florida plant killed him. In the process of trying to start the first subdivision in the Charlotte Harbor area with 200 priests, farmers, and artisans, he was summarily routed out by the existing residents, the Calusa Indians. During the attack, Ponce de León was injured by a poison-tipped Calusa arrow. The poison hailed from the sap of the manchineel tree, also known as the beach apple, with which the Calusa created rudimentary but highly effective biological weapons. Ponce de León fled to Cuba, where he soon died of the wound, never seeing his fiftieth birthday.

Ponce de León endowed us with our flowery name not out of any real appreciation for Florida's native beauty, although things were obviously in bloom at the time, but because he arrived at Easter, the Spanish *Pascua Florida*, or Festival of Flowers. It's not hard to imagine he may have perceived the floral landscape he encountered as confirmation of his divine right to take over, hubris of tragic dimensions.

Explorer and naturalist William Bartram, on the other hand, touring Florida in 1774, could barely contain his admiration for the world around him, enthusing, "O thou Creator supreme, almighty! how infinite and incomprehensible thy works! most perfect, and every way astonishing!"[1]

Florida delighted and amazed Bartram, as did almost every other place he visited, and he waxed especially eloquent over plants. "Perhaps there is not any part of creation, within the reach of our observations," he wrote, "which exhibits a more glorious display of the Almighty hand, than the vegetable world. Such a variety of pleasing scenes, ever changing, throughout the seasons, arising from various causes and assigned each to the purpose and use determined."[2]

He described in minute and prosaic detail our flora and fauna in his seminal work, *Travels through North & South Carolina, Georgia, East & West Florida*. He reveled in every careful step of his journey through Florida, writing of traveling over "fertile eminences and delightful, shady, fragrant forests," crossing "vivid green grassy turf," and passing "through fruitful orange groves. . . . level, open airy pine forest, the stately trees scatteringly planted by nature, arising straight and erect from the green carpet."[3]

He was attacked by alligators and hazarded by weather and Indian wars, but if he was at odds with anything or anyone in the landscape, he never let on. William Bartram died in 1823, strolling in his garden. He was 84.

Now, another 250 years down the road, even though it's a very different Florida than either Ponce de León or Bartram experienced, we're faced with similar prospects: resist and try to change our environment, or adapt and live in harmony with nature. Let's go with the premise that knowledge and understanding are far better guardians of health and well-being than fear and loathing.

The types of problematic human-plant interactions we're looking at in this section are contact allergies (phytodermatitis), respiratory allergies, oral allergies, and regional food allergies. But a little knowledge can go a long way toward keeping us safe and happy in our garden of Eden. A lot of the same Florida plants that can be harmful or provoke discomfort can also be quite beautiful or tasty or provide shelter for other animals and improve our environment.

So pull on your gardening gloves and blouse your pants. We're going for a hike.

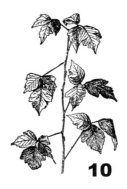

10

Look but Don't Touch

On every stem, on every leaf, . . . and at the root of everything that grew, was a professional specialist in the shape of grub, caterpillar, aphid, or other expert, whose business it was to devour that particular part.

Oliver Wendell Holmes

Rooted in place, soft, pliable, and seemingly passive, plants lie squarely at the bottom of a massive food chain. Everything, it seems, wants a piece of them: birds, animals, insects, and people. Without teeth or claws, plants must produce passive defenses, from a prickly armor of spines or hairs to toxic sap. Like insects, plants are unable to determine whether an accidental assailant, human or otherwise, is friend or foe. Everything and everyone gets the same treatment. For many who encounter plants' defensive weapons, that often amounts to phytodermatitis.

Understanding Phytodermatitis

Phytodermatitis is the medical term for skin reactions caused by plants. While specific statistics about phytodermatitis are hard to come by, the Asthma and Allergy Foundation of American (AAFA) reports that about 7 percent of those with allergies identify skin allergies—atopic dermatitis, eczema, hives, urticaria, and contact allergies—as their main complaint. Further, the American Academy of Allergy, Asthma and Immunology (AAAAI) says that skin allergies result in nearly 6 million doctor visits annually.

Those most commonly afflicted with phytodermatitis are people who occupationally work with plants, like farmers and agricultural workers, food handlers, caterers, grocers, florists, foresters, and landscapers. But weekend gardeners, hikers, bird-watchers, and hunters can have run-ins with less than friendly plants, too. As with most allergic reactions, some people exhibit more sensitivity than others. Those with fair hair and light skin, especially if they have existing pollen allergies, are generally more likely to experience some form of phytodermatitis than darker complexioned and dark-haired individuals. And younger children can easily become sensitized after a single exposure.[1]

Just as there are ways to identify plants most likely to cause inhalant allergies, there are also some specific clues to help identify plants that can cause skin contact problems. Author and botanist Thomas Ogren's allergen rating system, OPALS, which ranks plants from least allergenic (1) to most allergenic (10) can also be helpful with discussions about phytodermatology, and plants mentioned throughout will be identified with a parenthetical corresponding OPALS number, where available.

Here are some of the more distinguishing (or incriminating) features of plants most likely to cause phytodermatitis:

- Plants belong to certain botanical families, like cashew, olive, lily, or sunflower
- Plants with a milky sap
- Plants with spiky or hairy leaves or stems or with pollen grains having sharp "spines"
- Plants with numerous small flowers
- Plants with a disagreeable odor
- Any plant that causes an initial rash that is long lasting, severe, or scarring

The last one may seem obvious, but people sometimes exhibit a surprising inability to make connections; if touching a plant produces a rash or conjunctivitis (eye irritation) upon rubbing the eyes, the plant should be avoided in the future.

Most phytodermatitis symptoms occur, as might be expected, along the legs, arms, hands, and face. Dermatitis triggered by plants can be streaky in appearance, marking where skin brushed along a plant, and can produce redness, swelling, and sometimes blisters. If the rash is allergenic in nature, each subsequent contact will result in worsening reactions.

The list of plants that cause phytodermatitis is considerable, and there are several excellent books available on the topic with respect to gardening and landscaping, like Thomas Ogren's *Safe Sex in the Garden* and *Allergy-Free Gardening*. But there are few resources available for all-purpose outdoor recreation identification.

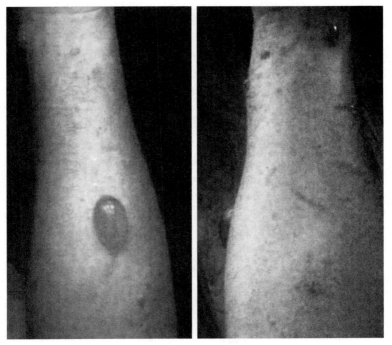

Urushiol-induced contact dermatitis on arms after 72 hours of contact with poison ivy. (Photo by Larsonja.)

So for our purposes here, we're going to look at some of the main allergy-causing agents and the principal families of plants that can produce the various types of contact dermatitis. And we'll look at them in the context of where they're most likely to be encountered, not just in a residential yard but also in parks and other outdoor environments.

Agents of Irritation

While there are literally thousands of phytodermatitis-inducing plants, there are just a handful of significant plant components that produce most of the symptoms and effects of phytodermatitis. The ones most commonly encountered are urushiol, calcium oxalate, and turpene.

Urushiol is an oleoresin, an oily resin, compound found in plants of the Anacardiaceae family, especially toxicodendrons like poison ivy and poison oak (10). The name derives from the Japanese word *urushi,* for a type of lacquer refined from the sap of the kirushi tree and used in the production of traditional Asian lacquerwares. One of its distinguishing features is that it dries black.

Kidney stone sufferers may be familiar with calcium oxalate. The compound forms needle-shaped crystals and occurs naturally in a variety of leafy green vegetables, the consumption of which predisposes some people to kidney stones. It also occurs in common plants like philodendrons, pineapples, and daffodils.

Turpenes are hydrocarbons that constitute the essential oils in plants. Turpenes occur in citrus, celery, and the pine trees from which turpentine was historically produced.

Other major allergenic plant compounds include phorbol ester, thiocyanate, protoanemonin, and capsaicin, which most people know as the heat in a chili pepper.

Any of the above, or several other plant compounds and proteins, can provoke phytodermatitis in any of four ways.

About 20 percent of phytodermatitis responses are allergenic in nature; the rest are irritant reactions.[2] But there's a lot of overlap between the two. Many allergenic chemicals are also physically irritating; for instance, handling narcissus bulbs can produce reactions

Table 10.1. Phytodermatitis responses

Dermatitis type	Characteristics	Causes	Plant examples
Irritant contact dermatitis (ICD)	Not an allergic response, and usually confined to areas of contact; can include mild irritation, blistering, swelling, or tissue necrosis; reactions can and usually do affect anyone, occur within minutes or hours, and last anywhere from a few hours to a few days.	May be "mechanical" from punctures, cuts, or scrapes from plant thorns, spines, or irritating hair like bristles, or chemically induced from plant acids, enzymes, or calcium oxalate crystals.	Prickly pear cactus Pineapples Bamboo Rose thorns Agave Philodendron Pineapple Buttercup Chile peppers Mango
Contact urticaria (hives)	Can be non-immunological, causing localized swelling and itching and lasting up to a few hours, or immunological (IgE mediated), producing generalized swelling, and lasting a day or so.	Non-immunological contact urticaria is toxin induced. Immunological responses are caused by proteins and pollen in plants that often become worse with subsequent exposure.	Can include many of the plants that cause ICD, but most commonly associated with stinging nettles.
Allergic contact dermatitis	Classic IgE-mediated response that can be delayed up to 48 hours, producing eczema, hives, and itching that can last a week or more; reactions usually begin at the area of contact and spread from there.	Allergic contact dermatitis is caused by sensitivity to alkaloids and oils in plants.	Mostly Compositae family of plants, including poison ivy, chrysanthemums, dandelions, goldenrod.
Photo dermatitis (Phytophoto-dermatitis)	Non-immunological reaction usually consisting of darkening or reddening of the skin with linear streaks; onset usually takes a few hours and can last days to years.	Triggered by plant chemicals, usually psoralens and angelicins in sap, combined with ultraviolet light.	Celery Carrots Limes Figs Queen Anne's lace

Source: Gunjan M. Modi, Christy B. Doherty, Rajani Katta, and Ida F. Orengo, "Irritant Contact Dermatitis from Plants: Chemical Irritant Contact Dermatitis," *MedScape Today*, WebMD, 2009, http://www.medscape.com/viewarticle/706404_3.

from mechanical irritant contact dermatitis (ICD) as well as chemical responses to the calcium oxalate crystals in the bulbs. We'll take a look at some examples of each.

Mechanical Dermatitis: Plants with Weapons

Several varieties of Florida plants come equipped with protective features like thorns, spines, bristles, hairs (known as trichomes), or coarse leaves and stems that can puncture, cut, or abrade the skin. Plants commonly found in Florida that can produce mechanical dermatitis include ivies, prickly pear cactus, hollies, mulberry, bamboo, and blackberry.

It's no accident that some of the tastiest fruits, like the blackberry and cactus fruit, are among the best protected.

Hairy Plants

Some plants are more subtle in their mechanical defenses. These include

- holly trees, with their sharp, stiff leaves;
- saw palmettos;
- bamboo fibers;
- pineapples;
- figs, mulberry, and primrose trees with their irritant hairs;
- thistles and burrs.

All of these plants can cause pain or itching when the tiny hairs that protect stems, leaves, or fruits become embedded in the skin, as anyone can attest who has brushed off itchy fig hairs or stepped on a sand spur at the beach.

Prickly Pear Cactus (*Opuntia humifusa*) (2)

The prickly pear is a great example of the dual lives of phytodermatitis-inducing plants. There are nine prickly pear cactus species in Florida, each of them quite literally cautioning, "Don't touch me!" even as they are eminently useful plants. The prickly pear is the only widespread eastern cactus, occurring in fields, woods, and roadsides. It has lovely, showy yellow flowers and edible fruit, a valuable resource to birds and animals who eat both seeds and fruit in great abundance.[3]

Many people also enjoy prickly pear fruit, which when peeled, sliced, and sprinkled with lemon juice is described as pleasantly sweet and tangy, albeit challenging to eat, since the fruit is covered with a coat of fine urticating hairs. Traditionally, the fruit is accessed with heavy gloves, and the hairs are singed off. The fruit can also be used to make preserves. The young stems of the cactus are also edible, and the sap can be used as a hair conditioner.[4]

Because cactus harbors such an obvious threat, it's a fairly easy plant to avoid, although the occasional hiker, cross-country runner, or geocacher might blunder into a smaller prickly pear. While the large spines pose a painful hazard, it's the smaller barbed glochid spines that occur in patches throughout the cactus that are the real

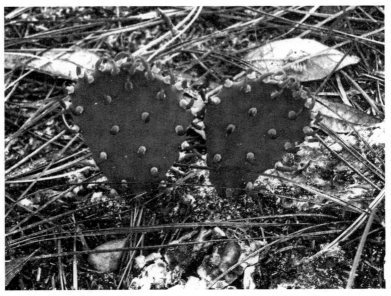

Prickly pear cactus. (Photo courtesy of Jeanene Arrington-Fisher, Not a Clue Adventures.)

danger, capable of producing "sabra dermatitis," as it's known in Israel where occupational cactus contact allergy is fairly common.

These smaller spines may not be immediately noticed while one is busy digging out the three-inch spines. But left in the skin, they can produce extensive and painful granular dermatitis that can persist for months. One efficient method of removing the glochids is to remove visible clumps of spines with tweezers and then apply household glue to the affected areas of skin. In studies, the dried glue, when peeled off, removed 95 percent of the spines.[5]

The Rose Family (Rosaceae) (OPALS vary by variety)

While the hazards of cultivated roses and of rose hips are well known, and there are some wild varieties in the state, hikers and outdoors people are far more likely to encounter its wild cousin, the bramble blackberry.

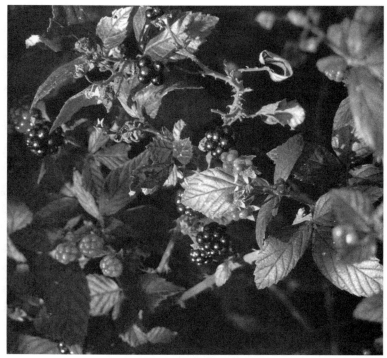

Wild blackberry bush. (Photo by Theresa Willingham.)

Blackberries grow wild throughout many Florida woodlands and fields. They're one of those dichotomous plants. Known as brambles for the almost impenetrable thorny thickets in which they grow, they're reviled by ranchers whose cattle can be injured by blackberry thorns and prized by blackberry lovers statewide.[6] Sometimes they can be reviled and loved at the same time, as when one is trying to pluck the fruit from its thorny stems, although gloves help considerably.

It's the unintentional encounters with blackberries that cause problems. Leaves have a fine coat of fuzzy hairs, and brambles snag shoes, socks, and pants. Blackberry thorn injuries promptly raise welts, and those hypersensitive to the abrasions (and whatever might be on the thorns) can suffer itching and hives.

Palm Trees (family Palmae or Arecaceae) (OPALS vary)

If you're not on personal terms with palm trees, the knowledge that some have thorns might come as a surprise. Pygmy date palms, commonly used in residential landscaping around the state, are particu-

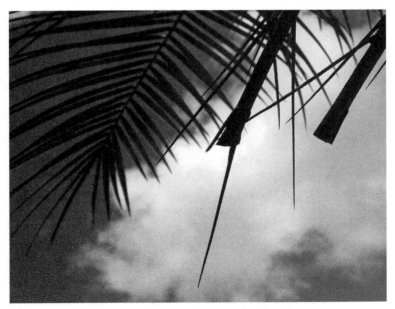

Pygmy date palm thorns. (Photo by Theresa Willingham.)

larly vicious, sporting thorns as long as three or four inches around the base of each frond. Trimming the palms, accidentally bumping into one of the spiky armed trees, or playing with cut fronds, which children may do, can result in some painful injuries that, without treatment, can produce infections, especially if the thorns pierce a joint area in the hands or knees.[7]

Medical literature abounds with an abundance of case references to arthritic-like conditions, usually synovitis (fluid collection in joints), and granulomas (tissue lesions) produced by palm thorn injuries. Even if palms don't have thorns, many have rough or bristly fronds that can irritate the skin on contact. The best way to avoid problems is to use thick gloves and to wear a hat and protective clothing when working with or near palm trees. Keep fiercely thorny species like the pygmy date palm away from areas where children play and away from walkways.

In treating a palm thorn injury, it's important to remove the thorn completely and clean the injured area thoroughly. If the thorn can't be removed or part of it breaks off in the skin, seek medical care.

Chemical Irritants: Plant Biological Warfare

Plants that cause chemical irritations do so with an arsenal of plant acids and enzymes. These chemical cocktails occur in some expected plants like chili peppers (from the Solanaceae, or nightshade family), and some possibly unexpected ones, like lilies (Cannaceae, or cana family) (4) and narcissus bulbs (Amaryllidaceae, or amaryllis family) (4), which can also cause contact urticaria, and the ubiquitous philodendron (Araceae, or arum family) (3). And the very components that can cause chemical contact dermatitis in some plants are also what make us value them, like the capsaicanoids that give chili peppers their bite and the thyiocynates that give mustard its flavor.[8]

Of Kidney Stones and Edema

Calcium oxalate is among the most common of the irritant compounds, found in varying concentrations in more than 200 plant families. The same needle-shaped crystals that produce kidney stones are thought to function as a protective mechanism in the plant for fending off foraging wildlife.

The common household plant, dieffenbachia (arum family) (5), also known as dumb cane for its ability to render those who chew its leaves hoarse or unable to speak, contains an abundance of calcium oxalate. While many plants that contain the chemical are also poisonous to ingest, the ones we're looking at cause contact dermatitis ranging from redness and itching to generalized edema.

Garden Warfare

Many of the plants we enjoy having in Florida gardens and landscapes can be as physically noxious as they are aesthetically pleasing. An extreme example is the oleander (Apocynaceae, or dogbane family) (6).

Blossoming in profusion along medians and right of ways throughout Florida, oleanders are among the most toxic of plants, containing a lethal cocktail of chemicals that produce everything from skin rashes on contact with sap to acute poisoning and cardiac arrest if ingested.

Typically, the most common culprits in chemically induced contact dermatitis are from plants that contain the aforementioned calcium oxalate, which is also found in daisies (Asteraceae/Compositae, the aster/daisy family) (6), dog fennel (*Eupatorium capillifolium*) (7), daffodils (related to narcissus) (4), and hyacinths (Liliaceae, the lily family) (3). Other problematic chemical compounds and the plants in which they occur include

- thiocyanates, in Allicaeae and Brassicaceae, or the spicy herbs;
- diterpene esters, most common in Euphorbiaceae, or the spurges, crotons (4), poinsettias, and castor bean plants (10); and
- protoanemonins, found in the family Ranunculaceae, which includes buttercups (5), crocus (2), and clematis (3).[9]

Most of these chemical compounds are found in these plants' sticky white latex sap, sometimes occurring throughout the plant and sometimes just in the leaves, stems, or bulbs.

"Tulip fingers" is a sometimes disfiguring condition that affects nursery workers routinely handling chemically irritating tulip bulbs for sorting or planting. "Daffodil itch" affects florists and nursery workers and is relatively confined to areas of contact and resolved when contact ceases.

Among the spices, garlic is the most common cause of fingertip dermatitis among both home and restaurant cooks. Fresh garlic (amaryllis family) (2), which can also produce allergies, is so potent an irritant that it can actually cause second and third degree burns if applied to injured skin.[10] "Flowering garlic" is also used as an ornamental plant in residential landscapes.

Most of the plants in the chemical irritant category are relatively easy to avoid or to protect against. Carefully selecting garden plants, if sensitivity is an issue, or wearing long sleeves and gloves while gardening usually provides sufficient protection against reactions.

Contact Urticaria

Irritant contact dermatitis (ICD) can range in presentation from mild irritation, redness, and swelling to tissue damage at the site of contact. Contact urticaria, on the other hand, presents as hives, sometimes extensive, consisting of dark red, swollen, itchy bumps that can appear anywhere on the skin, regardless of where contact occurred and whether the reaction is immunologic or not.[11]

People can experience urticaria to some degree as a result of casual contact with something that irritates the skin, from allergic reactions to bees or wasps or to seafood, or as nonallergic responses to sinusitis or food additives, or any number of things. I once experienced urticaria on both hands and parts of my arms. My hands turned red, itched, and swelled enormously. Antihistamines were prescribed, and after a few days the whole thing subsided. Neither I nor the immunologist was any wiser about what caused the urticaria in the first place.

Contact urticaria from plants is typically "toxin-mediated" or non-immunologic in nature, although immunologic contact urticaria can and does occur, sometimes as a result of cross-allergies. Celery (Apiaceae, the carrot family) (5) is the most common cause of plant-related immunologic contact urticaria. Fruits are also common triggers, including apples (4), peaches (3–4), plums (3) (all in the rose family), bananas (Musaceae) (5), oranges (Rutaceae, or citrus family) (3), and mangoes (Araceae, arum family) (10).[12]

Plants that are known to cause chemical irritant contact dermatitis, like garlic, tulips, and lilies, can also cause immunologic contact urticaria. If suspected, immunologic contact urticaria triggers can be identified through skin prick tests. Prevention is the best treatment, although keeping antihistamines on hand can help.

Toxin-mediated, or non-immunologic, contact urticaria is the most often encountered, though, and usually attributed, fittingly, to plants of the Urticaceae family, or the nettles. The word *urticaria*, in fact, stems from the Latin *urtica*, or nettle. And no nettle is more nettlesome than the stinging nettle.

Stinging Nettles (*Urtica dioica*) (10)

Stinging nettles are as unforgiving as their name suggests. A low-growing weedy herb common in flood plains, woods, disturbed areas, and farm yards, our family also discovered that it grows well at Disney World. Many years ago, when our middle daughter was about 6 years old, we were all enjoying the man-made waterfront at Ft. Wilderness with out-of-town friends, when she suddenly yelped and emerged crying from behind a large landscape boulder. She held out her hand, which was quickly reddening, and said that a plant had stung her.

Peering under the rock where she'd been digging, we saw a rather nondescript plant with scalloped leaves which a kindly Disney employee, rendering prompt first aid, identified as stinging nettle. That was the first and only time I've ever seen one, although we've been on the alert ever since.

Stinging nettles, it turns out, are an amorphous lot, varying in appearance according to where they're growing. Plants in shady areas have coarsely toothed leaves and weaker stems than plants growing in the open, which also have tighter flower clusters and look like tall

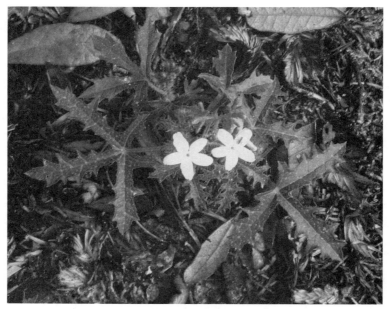

Stinging nettle. (Photo courtesy of Jeanene Arrington-Fisher, Not a Clue Adventures.)

parsley plants and sometimes like maple leaves. They can grow up to two feet high in open areas.

Regardless of appearance, all the stinging nettles feature stiff hollow stinging hairs along the stem and on leaves that, when broken, inject irritant histamines and acetocholines (a type of neurotransmitter) into the skin. While immediate, frightening, and intense, reactions are generally short-lived.[13]

More severe reactions are rare, and the plant is widely used to treat enlarged prostates, urinary tract infections, arthritis and allergic rhinitis.[14] Studies are also under way to explore the plant's use in lowering blood sugar and treating high blood pressure.

The plants aren't common in residential areas, but may be encountered while hiking or enjoying other outdoors activities. The best way to avoid them is to wear long pants while hiking, stay on cleared trails, and avoid reaching into unknown areas.

Treatment consists of removing the glochids, or stinging hairs, with tweezers, by washing, or repeatedly applying tape to which the hairs can adhere. Washing the area promptly and applying a baking soda paste or calamine lotion usually relieves the stinging fairly promptly, as it did for our daughter. A few unrelated varieties of stinging plants include spurges known as the bull nettle or spurge nettles, encounters with which are similarly treated and avoided.

Allergic Contact Dermatitis

Allergic contact dermatitis is a classic IgE-mediated response that can occur within two days of contact with the allergen and can produce eczema, hives, and itching that lasts a week or more. Reactions may begin at the area of contact, but may spread extensively. The most common culprits in allergic contact dermatitis are plants in the Anacardiaceae, or sumac, family, especially those in the genus *Toxicodendron*, which contain urushiol.

The Toxicodendrons (10)

Almost anyone who's been outdoors in Florida (and most wilderness areas throughout the United States) can probably describe the basics of the best known of the toxicodendrons, poison ivy, beginning with that useful childhood mnemonic, "Leaves of three leave it be." While lots of other nontoxic plants have "leaves of three," the old adage is a tried and true rule of thumb that can help keep children, and adults, out of harm's way.

And there's plenty of harm to be had. Florida has three species of toxicodendrons: poison ivy, poison oak, and poison sumac.

Poison ivy grows as a vine that can reach 10 feet in length, often climbing along trees, walls, or houses. All parts of the plant are poisonous.[15]

Poison oak, despite its name, isn't a tree but a shrub with oaklike leaves; otherwise, it is almost indistinguishable from poison ivy. It grows along disturbed areas by roads, trails, and stream banks.

Poison sumac possesses seven to thirteen leaflets per each reddish leaf and can grow to be much larger than its cousins, occurring as a shrub or small tree that can range from 5 to 25 feet in height.

The principal irritating component in all three is urushiol. On

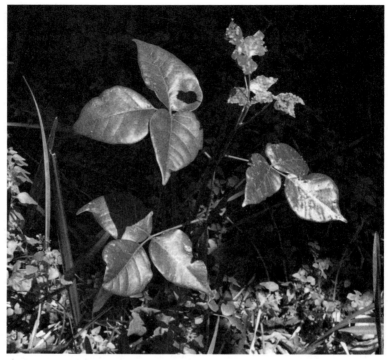

Poison ivy. (Photo by Theresa Willingham.)

contact with skin, the sap of toxicodendron plants can produce an autoimmune response ranging from itching to redness, streaking, inflammation, blisters, and severe burning sensations. Some people develop "black-spot poison-ivy dermatitis," so called for the black spot that forms over the blisters. But prompt washing seems to reduce the chances of this form of dermatitis.

The sap is tenacious and will continue to cause reactions on contact wherever it adheres, whether on skin, clothing, tents, or shoes, until it is washed off.

Toxicodendrons can also produce throat and eye irritation and skin rashes when the plants are burned. Burning poison ivy can pose a serious threat to firefighters as well as to campers, who may inadvertently burn poison ivy and related plants with campfire tinder and inhale the urushiol-laden smoke.

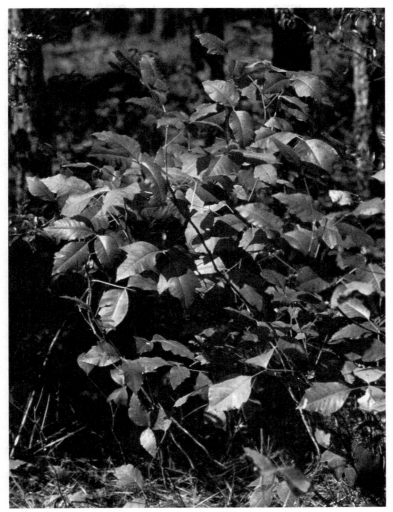

Atlantic poison oak. (Photo by James H. Miller, USDA Forest Service, Bugwood.org. Creative Commons Attribution 3.0 License.)

Poison Ivy Treatments

Without any treatment, rashes typically resolve themselves within a couple of weeks and usually leave no scars. However, excessive scratching can cause secondary infections that may require antibi-

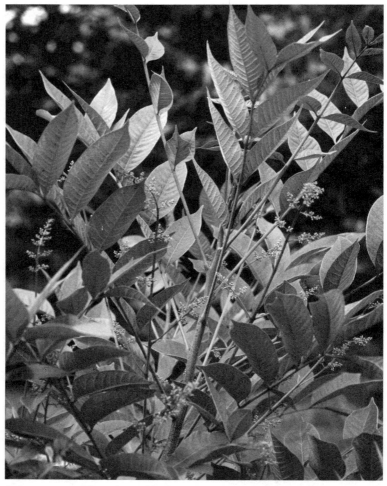

Poison sumac. (Photo by Ted Bodner, Southern Weed Science Society, Bugwood.org. Creative Commons Attribution 3.0 License.)

otic treatments, so it's helpful to alleviate itching with antihistamines and topical treatments.

Several products are marketed for the removal of urushiol saps from clothing and skin and to treat rashes more effectively. One study looked at two over-the-counter treatments and compared them with household dishwashing liquid in washing off poison ivy.

Researchers found that the pharmacy treatments weren't as effective as advertised and only a little more effective than the dishwashing liquid, which offered up to 60 percent protection against the urushiol for far less money.[16] Immunotherapy has also not proven effective against poison ivy allergy.

Here are a few other tips:

- Fluid from poison ivy blisters does not spread poison ivy, although urushiol can be spread upon early contact to other parts of the body.[17]
- Wash promptly after contact, preferably with some type of solvent, like rubbing alcohol or acetone, which will help remove the oily sap from your skin, and then rinse thoroughly with water. Plain soap and cold water may do the trick, too, if applied within a few minutes of contact.
- Apply ice to reduce itching and discomfort. Thomas Ogren reports applications of apple cider vinegar can also be effective.
- Wash clothes thoroughly.
- Wash any garden tools, shoes, or hiking equipment that may have come into contact with poison ivy.

Other Allergenic Anacardiaceae

Many other plants in the Anacardiaceae family can cause allergic contact dermatitis. Some, like the cashew nut tree and mango, which both rank 10 on OPALS, occur mostly in home landscaping environments. Others, like the poisonwood tree and Brazilian pepper (7–10), might be encountered on outdoor hikes or in the course of other outdoor recreation. Interestingly, the cashew, mango, and Brazilian pepper, all imports from Latin America, don't cause allergic dermatitis there with the frequency that they do in the United States.[18]

Cashew Tree (*Anacardium occidentale*)(10)

The cashew tree, also known as cashew apple, is Brazilian in origin but grows easily throughout much of the tropics, and quite well in South Florida where it is a prized evergreen shade and fruit tree. Its gifts come with considerable caveats, though.

According to the University of Florida IFAS Extension Service, nuts from landscape trees shouldn't be harvested for consumption by homeowners because both the nutshell and the tree sap contain potent allergens. The oil from the nutshell can actually cause extensive blistering, and even cashew flowers can cause dermatitis.

Mango (*Mangifera indica L*) (10)

The mango is a much beloved fruit in Florida. Mangoes are seasonally available in grocery stores around the state. They're also highly allergenic for some people.

There are about 35 species of mango worldwide. Two grow in Florida. The Indian mango is commercially grown here, whereas the Indochinese and hybridized varieties occur mostly in home landscapes. Like the toxicodendrons, the cut or peeled skin of mango fruits contains urushiol—not as much as poison ivy, but in concentrations high enough to produce allergic contact dermatitis in some people.

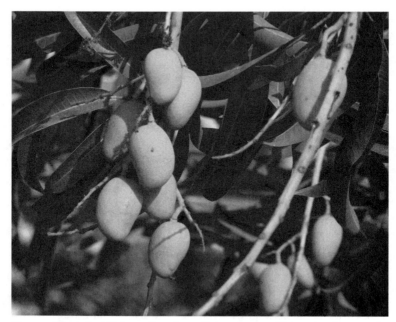

Mango. (Photo by Whitney Cranshaw, Colorado State University, Bugwood. org. Creative Commons Attribution 3.0 License.)

Those sensitive to mangoes will experience symptoms similar to that caused by a run-in with poison ivy, including hives and blisters. There is some evidence that people with existing sensitivity to toxicodendrons may be predisposed, or cross-reactive, to mango contact allergy.[19]

All parts of the mango can produce contact allergy symptoms, including the skin, leaves, stem, and bark of the plant. In addition to urushiol, mango also contains the phenol cardol, a component of cashews as well. Peeling the fruit (and washing promptly after doing so) helps prevent contact dermatitis, and the fruit itself is typically not as allergenic, although some people are sensitive to that as well.[20]

Brazilian Pepper (*Schinus terebinthifolius*) (7–10)

Sometimes erroneously identified as Florida holly, the Brazilian pepper is neither from Florida, nor a holly tree, but rather the scourge of native Florida woodlands. There are, in fact, eleven species of native holly in Florida including the landscape favorite, the dahoon holly,

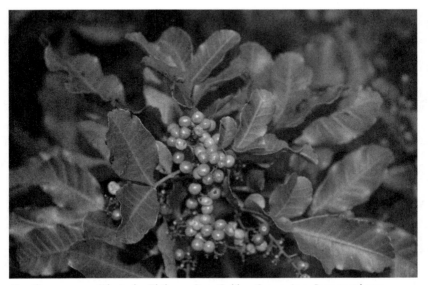

Brazilian pepper. (Photo by Zhihong Pan, Galileo Group, Inc., Bugwood.org. Creative Commons Attribution 3.0 License.)

and none of them are allergenic beyond an occasional poke from their sharp-tipped leaves.

Hundreds of volunteers labor year-round to remove the aggressive and tenacious invasive Brazilian pepper from parks and preserves statewide. Add to its pernicious character the fact that it also can produce allergic contact dermatitis and there's just very little nice to say about this ubiquitous and stubborn plant.

It was imported to the state in the mid-1800s as an ornamental, presumably because none of our thousands of native trees were decorative enough for Victorian Floridians. It is unfortunate that the tree is such a hit with wildlife, especially birds, which spread Brazilian pepper seeds widely throughout the state and compound the problem.

Most parts of the plant can cause allergic contact dermatitis as well as inflammation of the face and eyes. Contact with the cambrium, the live-tissue layer just beneath the bark of the tree, can cause a severe rash. In addition, the flowers and fruits can cause respiratory problems, and allergic rhinitis can occur in people pruning or cutting down Brazilian pepper, especially when it's flowering. The berries are toxic to ingest.

Anyone working with Brazilian pepper is advised to wear gloves and protective clothing. And for the record, Brazilian pepper is an official "noxious weed" in Florida, making it illegal to possess and cultivate it anywhere in the state.[21]

Poisonwood Tree (*Metopium toxiferum*)

The poisonwood tree, also known as the hog gum, is found mostly in the Florida Keys, but also occurs in hardwood hammocks around South Florida. It grows as an evergreen shrub or a medium-sized tree, reaching up to 35 feet in height. It's most identifying characteristic is its thin reddish-brown or gray bark spotted with dark, oily patches of gummy sap. All parts of the tree can cause allergic contact dermatitis. As hazardous as the plant is to people, it serves as an important food source for the endangered white crowned pigeon, which only lives in the Florida Keys and South Florida.[22]

Fickle Flowers

While not responsible for allergic contact dermatitis to the degree or frequency of Anacardiaceae, plants from the families Asteraceae or Compositae can also cause problems. The garden of this second-largest family of flowering plants, alternately known as the aster (6–8), daisy (6–7), or sunflower family (5), is also responsible for a high number of food allergies as well as cross-reactive problems.

One of the main allergenic plants from this family is the dandelion (6). Used medicinally worldwide as a mild diuretic and immune system booster, and usually considered safe, the latex sap of the plant can cause allergic contact dermatitis, especially if an individual is also allergic to their Asteraceae cousins ragweed (10), chrysanthemums (4–7), marigold (6), chamomile (7), yarrow (7), or daisies (6–7), or to iodine.[23]

The main culprits in Asteraceae allergies are compounds called sesquiterpene lactones. Sensitivity is more common among those handling plants like mums and marigolds occupationally but can also occur among residential gardeners and anyone casually encountering the flowers.[24]

Sunflowers can also cause allergic contact dermatitis among those harvesting plants and seeds for consumption and landscaping. Sunflower plant trichomes, the tiny hairs on stems and leaves, especially when dislodged in dry plant material, seem to be the major culprit in this case.

Herby Hives

Plants of the family Alliaceae, genus *Allium*, consisting of onions, garlic and chives, and previously implicated in chemical contact dermatitis, can also provoke allergic contact dermatitis in sensitive individuals. Garlic is the most common cause of allergic contact dermatitis in this group. To a far lesser degree, mints, sage, and thyme can also trigger allergic contact dermatitis.

Treatment

While not widely used to treat allergic contact dermatitis to Compositae plants, immunotherapy has shown some success. The principal evidence for the benefits of hyposensitization is the fact that while chrysanthemum allergy is the most common Compositae allergy in Europe, it's rare in Japan where the leaves and flowers are routinely eaten.[25] Topical ointments and oral antihistamines are only effective if taken early after exposure.

Photochemotherapy (PUVA)—ironically utilizing a component that can trigger phytophotodermatitis—has been helpful in treating Compositae dermatitis, especially in combination with prednisone. But the best treatment remains preventing contact in the first place.

Phytophotodermatitis

If Adam really wore a fig leaf in the Garden of Eden, he was flirting with a truly uncomfortable case of phytophotodermatitis (PPD). This is a Rube Goldberg kind of chemical reaction in the body: contact with compounds in certain plants makes the skin sensitive to ultraviolet (UV) light, which is basically sunlight. The condition manifests itself within 24 hours of exposure to a sensitizing plant, producing reddening of the skin with a burning sensation like sunburn and sometimes blistering. Pigmentary changes in the skin can result, which sometimes actually resemble burns and can vary in severity.[26]

The plants commonly causing PPD are those in the Apiaceae, or Umbelliferae, family, consisting of aromatic, hollow-stemmed herbal perennials like parsley, dill, fennel, and parsnips, collectively known as umbellifers. The culprit is a compound in the plants called psoralen, which is used in the treatment of skin disorders like psoriasis, eczema, and vitiligo as well as in tanning accelerators.[27]

Other plants that can produce PPD include citrus, legumes (peas and beans), mulberry (10, males), and figs. Certain occupations, hobbies, and situations may predispose someone to acquiring PPD:

- Agricultural work, either commercial or domestic
- Outdoor recreation in grass or fields containing umbellifers like Queen Anne's lace
- Occupations involving regular contact with limes or celery, such as bartending or restaurant work
- Use of commercial or home tanning beds after eating excessively of foods that contain psoralens

Treating PPD

Once the problem is identified, PPD flare-ups can be treated with a combination of topical corticosteroids and cold wet compresses to reduce discomfort. Prevention consists of avoiding contact with the plants that cause PPD.

In Summary

- Phytodermatitis refers to skin reactions caused by contact with certain plants.
- There are four basic types of phytodermatitis: (1) irritant contact dermatitis (ICD), either mechanical or chemical; (2) contact urticaria (hives); (3) allergic contact dermatitis; and (4) phytophotodermatitis (light sensitivity).
- Phytodermatitis reactions can include localized or generalized eczema, conjunctivitis, itching, redness, and swelling.
- About 20 percent of phytodermatitis responses are allergenic in nature; the rest are irritant reactions.
- Phytodermatitic plants often belong to the sumac, cashew, olive, lily, or sunflower families and have marked characteristics, such as milky sap, hairy plant parts, or numerous small flowers, among other features.
- Ranking plants on a scale of 1 to 10 from least to most allergenic, the Ogren Plant Allergy Scale (OPALS) is a helpful tool for identifying the allergy potential of certain plants.
- Mechanical irritant contact dermatitis can be caused by prickly pear cactus, saw palmettos, pygmy date palms, holly trees, roses, blackberries, and sandspurs.

- Chemical irritant contact dermatitis is most commonly caused by plants that contain calcium oxalate, thiocyanates, diterpene esters, and protoanemonins. These can include dieffenbachia and philodendron, spice and herb plants like garlic and onions, plants from the lily and daffodil groups, as well as crotons, poinsettias, and oleanders.
- Contact urticaria presents as hives anywhere on the skin, regardless of where contact occurred or whether the reaction is immunologic or non-immunologic. Celery is the most common culprit, but contact urticaria can also be caused by mangoes, bananas, oranges, apples, peaches, and plums.
- Stinging nettles are the most common cause of non-immunologic (or toxin-mediated) contact urticaria.
- Allergic contact dermatitis, an IgE-mediated response, may be delayed by up to two days and can produce eczema, hives, and itching that lasts a week or more. Though most commonly caused by plants in the toxicodendron, or sumac, family—poison ivy, poison oak, and poison sumac—it is also caused by the Florida poisonwood tree, the cashew apple, the Brazilian pepper, the mango, and plants from the Compositae family including sunflowers and dandelions and herbal plants like onions, garlic, and chives.
- Phytophotodermatitis (PPD) is a chemical reaction caused by the compound psoralen in certain plants, which makes skin sensitive to ultraviolet (UV) light. Skin irritation resembles sunburn, sometimes accompanied by blistering and pigmentary changes. Plants in the Umbelliferae family, like parsley, dill, fennel, and parsnips, are the most common cause of PPD.
- Phytodermatitis may be prevented by (1) wearing appropriate clothing outdoors; (2) not touching the face (especially the eyes) when engaged in outdoor activities; (3) using female landscape plants; (4) showering promptly after being outdoors; and (5) laundering clothes thoroughly.

11

Stop to Smell the Roses
but Take Shallow Breaths

A flower's appeal is in its contradictions—so delicate in form yet
strong in fragrance, so small in size yet big in beauty, so short in life
yet long on effect.

Terri Guillemets

We've discussed seasonal pollen allergies, largely with respect to trees
and grasses, but some people can suffer from nonseasonal flower
and plant allergies or from "nonallergic vasomotor rhinitis," both
discomforts worth mentioning. The latter is a mouthful, but if your
nose starts running when you get a whiff of strong perfumes, ciga-
rette smoke, or other overpowering scents, you've experienced nonallergic rhinitis.

Nonallergic reactions are important because they can often be the
triggers for true allergic responses that can be more problematic.[1]
And they also occur pretty regularly in a lot of people.

This chapter will explore the various plants that can cause respiratory distress, sometimes seasonally, like oak trees and grasses,
and sometimes not. And we'll look at how to reduce exposure and
symptoms and how to create allergy-free gardens and flower arrangements.

Nonseasonal Allergic Rhinitis

As we learned in the first section, in some people, inhaling pollen from plants to which they're sensitive triggers a release of histamines, prostaglandins, and leukotrienes that can cause congestion, respiratory difficulty, itching, and irritability. While the most common culprits are the seasonal anemophilous, or "wind-pollinated," plants like oak and mulberry trees, grasses and ragweeds, a few brightly flowered entomophilous, or "insect-pollinated," plants like daisies, dahlias, sunflowers, and sometimes even roses can produce pollen allergies any time of the year.[2]

The problem can occur in flower gardens and with indoor plants in homes and workplaces that may flower at nonspecific times. And some inhalant allergies can occur to plants that don't even produce pollen. OPALS ratings are referenced where available.

Indoor Plant Allergies

In a 2006 study of people suffering from allergic rhinitis, nearly 80 percent proved sensitive to indoor plants. The study looked at the common ornamentals yucca (2), ivy (7/8 in outdoor varieties), palm trees, geraniums (3), and ficus (2), or weeping fig—almost all present to some degree in homes, offices, and buildings throughout Florida. In addition to rhinitis, nearly 40 percent experienced intermittent asthma, 32 percent had conjunctivitis, and 12 percent suffered from dermatitis. The ficus, while relatively low on the allergy scale, proved the most allergenic of the indoor plants in the study.[3]

The weeping fig, or *Ficus benjamina*, is an exotic import that thrives indoors and out in Florida. It can reach heights of up to 60 feet and grow as big as 60 to 70 feet across, especially in South Florida, where conditions for it are ideal. But allergenic problems to the plant appear to occur principally indoors.

In the study, researchers theorized that people sensitive to the ficus inhale the components of its milky sap, which is diffused from the plant's leaves and becomes airborne when mixed with indoor dust.[4] Other studies suggest sensitivity to *Ficus benjamina*, as an indoor household allergen, may be as common as allergy to mold.[5]

Ficus allergy can produce cross-reactivity to latex, too.[6] Additionally, houseplants can create welcoming environments for mold, which can cause problems for those sensitive to mold spores.

Flower Power

While it's usually true that bright, colorful flowers rarely cause allergies, compared with paler varieties, several types of flowers can cause pollen-related allergic reactions. Members of the Asteraceae/Compositae families commonly used in household and special event bouquets like daisies (6), gerbera (6), chrysanthemums (4–7), asters (6–8), dahlias (6), and sunflowers (5), as well as lilies (4) from the amaryllis family, are the most common culprits, particularly those of the "single" flowered type.[7]

Allergies to colorful flowers are normally rare because the plants that produce brightly colored flowers are typically insect-pollinated rather than wind-pollinated, and their pollen is consequently better contained within the flower. In household or other indoor use, however, colorful flowers are handled, shaken, and sniffed, with the result that pollen is shaken free into the air and inhaled.

Pollen-free flower varieties known as "formal doubles" solve that problem in an attractive way, with petal-like "staminoids"—basically a pollen-less stamen—and lots of petals per flower. There are now several formal double varieties of chrysanthemums, dahlias, and asters that are truly allergy-free.[8]

Diagnosing, Treating, and Preventing Indoor Plant Allergy

Indoor plant allergies can be diagnosed in the same way as outdoor allergies, via allergy testing. Treatment for mild allergic responses include the usual over-the-counter antihistamines and corticosteroids as well as immunotherapy.

Once an allergy to indoor plants is discovered, the easiest solution is to remove them from the home. Silk plants are one solution, although they can collect dust and cause other problems for those sensitive to airborne allergens. Another solution is to use low-allergy indoor plants like the following:

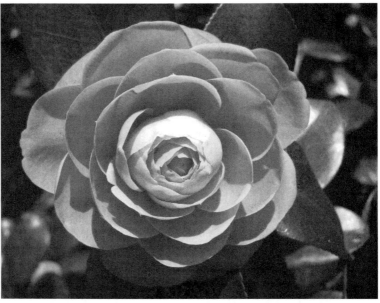

Pollen-free double camellia blossom. (Photo by Rebekah D. Wallace, Bugwood.org. Creative Commons Attribution 3.0 License.)

- Orchids (family Orchidaceae) (1)
- African violets (family Gesneriaceae) (1)
- Camellias (1 for double blossom varieties)
- Cacti (1/2), like the lovely Christmas cactus
- Jade plant (*Crassula ovate*) (2)
- Pansies and violas (family Violaceae) (1) and impatiens (1), not really indoor plants but able to thrive in a sunny Florida room.

In flower arrangements, special low- or no-pollen varieties of roses like Cecile Brunner and Banksia are good choices, as are orchids, hydrangea, begonias (2), and camellias.

Nonallergic Rhinitis (NAR)

Anyone who's had the eye-watering companionship of a heavily perfumed seatmate on an airplane or in a restaurant is familiar with

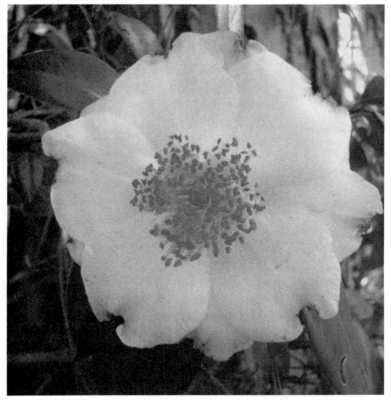

Single blossom camellia, with more prominent stamen and consequent pollen. (Photo by Rebekah D. Wallace, Bugwood.org. Creative Commons Attribution 3.0 License.)

nonallergic rhinitis, or NAR. Also known as "vasomotor rhinitis"— dilation of the blood vessels in the nose—this condition produces congestion, runny nose, itching, and other symptoms without the allergy.

Ruling out true allergies and things like sinus infections, nasal polyps, or a deviated septum, any number of things can cause the nasal inflammation of vasomotor rhinitis.[9]

- Environmental irritants like smog, secondhand smoke, chemical fumes or perfumes, and "sick building syndrome"

- Changes in temperature or humidity
- Viral infections
- Consumption of hot or spicy foods or alcohol
- Medications, like nonsteroidal anti-inflammatory drugs (NSAIDS), or beta-blockers
- Hormonal changes
- Stress

There are also several factors that increase the risk of vasomotor rhinitis.

- Occupational exposure to irritants
- Overuse of decongestant nasal treatments
- Gender—women tend more toward nonallergic rhinitis than men
- Asthma, lupus, or other medical conditions

With respect to Florida, the things that can cause nonallergic rhinitis include

- environmental changes produced by going between our hot and humid outdoors and cold, dry air-conditioned indoors;
- smoke, including muck fires and woodsy southern bar-beques; and
- fragrant flowers.

It's thought that anywhere from 23 to 70 percent of adults experience NAR, for which most seek treatment from general practitioners rather than allergists.

The condition is significant beyond the annoyance factor because studies confirm that regular bouts of NAR can evolve into full blown allergic rhinitis when sufferers become sensitized to airborne allergens.[10] As a matter of fact, fully half of seasonal allergy sufferers report that their symptoms are triggered by extreme temperature changes and smoke.[11]

Muck Fires

We're no California, but every year we have our share of wildfires. "Muck" fires are a particularly odiferous variety indigenous to Florida, and they occur when swampy or marshy areas ignite during dry season due to careless smokers, lightning strikes, and, some might say, spontaneous combustion. Muck fires are actually underground conflagrations within layers of peat and can burn as deep as 500 feet underground and produce a withering smolder for weeks or even months.

Smoke from muck fires can be impenetrable and can literally take the breath away, causing stinging eyes, breathing difficulties, and rhinitis. Young children and the elderly are most at risk for smoke-related NAR, but anyone sensitive to smoke and strong odors can be affected.

The best way to avoid problems is to avoid going outside when there are fires, which typically occur during the drier late winter and spring months. News reports will usually advise of fire-related weather conditions. For those who must go out when fires are burning, wearing a dust particle mask can help.

Fragrant Flowers

Like temperature, smoke, and spicy foods, fragrant flowers can cause NAR symptoms for some people, especially strongly perfumed flowers like gardenias (4), with their deep and heady fragrance, and jasmine (7), particularly the strongly aromatic night-blooming variety. Jasmine pollen is also highly allergenic to some people, so an initial NAR experience could easily morph into allergic rhinitis.

Here are other heavily fragrant flowers that can induce vasomotor rhinitis:

- Lilac (6)
- Alyssum (6)
- Magnolia (5/6), especially *Magnolia acuminata*, also known as "cucumbertree"
- Citrus blossoms (4–5)
- Plumeria (frangipani)(4)
- Lilies (4)
- Butterfly ginger (5)
- Honeysuckle (5)
- Dianthus (3)
- Roses (OPALS varies by variety)

Aromatic spices and herbs like pepper, onion (2), and garlic (2) can also trigger NAR, either as fresh growing flowers and plants or in their dried forms.

It's interesting to note that most of the heavily aromatic flowers that can induce nonallergic rhinitis are also often implicated in more straightforward pollen or contact dermatitis–related allergies.

Treating and Preventing NAR

Nonallergic rhinitis is diagnosed by ruling out other sinus problems, usually via a nasal endoscopy or CT scan, as well as by testing for suspected allergenic triggers. If results to those tests are negative, then vasomotor rhinitis is usually the safe assumption.

Treatment varies by severity of the problem. For those only mildly bothered by strong odors or fumes, treatment consists of avoiding or ameliorating conditions like temperature extremes that can trigger a reaction. But there are also some health practices that may prove helpful, like the unpleasant sounding but apparently effective practice of "nasal lavage," or nasal irrigation, using warm saltwater or sodium bicarbonate mixtures. (Check with a physician for proper technique.)[12]

Other helpful practices include blowing the nose regularly and gently when in the presence of irritants, using a humidifier at work or at home, especially in sleeping quarters, staying hydrated, and avoiding caffeine, which can lead to dehydration and exacerbate NAR symptoms. Over-the-counter treatments include oral or spray decongestants, saline nasal sprays, and antihistamines.

If none of these prove helpful, a physician may prescribe more effective medications. As usual, though, prevention is the best treatment, and staying away from strongly aromatic flowers, if that's the main trigger, is the best solution.

NAR-Free Flowers

Many of the same flowers that are safe for those with allergic rhinitis are also good for those with vasomotor rhinitis. Plants like orchids, African violets, and jade plants are beautiful and low impact with respect to rhinitis symptoms. Other plants that can be included in flower arrangements or outdoor gardens include impatiens (1), snapdragons (1), phlox (4), peonies (2), and petunias (2). In flower arrangements, closed bud tea roses, hydrangea, begonias, and camellias are good choices.

In Summary

- In addition to seasonal pollen allergies, some people suffer from nonseasonal plant allergies and from vasomotor (nonallergic) rhinitis.
- Common indoor ornamental plants like ivy, yucca, potted palms, and ficus (especially the "weeping fig" variety) have been found to aggravate existing allergic conditions.
- There is evidence that asthma can be aggravated by indoor plant allergies.
- "Double formal" pollen-free or low pollen–producing flower varieties are a good choice for those with flower allergies, as are orchids, African violets, and other 1 and 2 OPALS-rated flowers and plants.
- Flower allergies are diagnosed and treated in the same way as other IgE-mediated allergic reactions.
- Nonallergic rhinitis, or NAR, is an allergy-like response to strong odors or fumes. Common NAR triggers are extreme temperature changes, smoke, spices, and strong aromas from perfumes or flowers.
- Florida flowers that commonly cause NAR include fragrant gardenias, jasmine, lilies, frangipani, citrus blossoms, and honeysuckle.
- Nonallergic rhinitis is diagnosed by ruling out true allergies and sinus problems.
- NAR treatments vary by severity of the problem and range from simply avoiding the stimulus to use of over-the-counter nasal sprays and decongestants.
- Low-aroma flowers like orchids, African violets, and camellias are good choices for those with NAR symptoms.

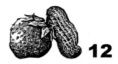 **12**

Why Does My Tongue Itch?

Nature cannot be tricked or cheated. She will give up to you
the object of your struggles only after you have paid her price.

Napoleon Hill

We've examined a variety of inhalant and contact plant irritants, including pollens, chemical and mechanical irritants, and aromatic sensitivities. Now we're going to get down to the business of eating.

Since almost everything and anything can grow here, Florida has an enormous range of culinary delights, homegrown and imported, in which to indulge and also from which to suffer if you have food sensitivities. Food allergies form a huge subject all by themselves, and there are plenty of treatises on the topic, including my own *Food Allergy Field Guide*.[1] Our focus here, however, is on the ethnobotany of the Sunshine State.

In addition to seasonally available products like our citrus and other familiar fruits and vegetables found nationwide (and often grown right here, one of the nation's most productive agricultural regions), Florida features some homegrown specialties like avocados, carambola, coconuts, mangoes, lychees, and papayas.

Some, like coconut, can produce outright food allergies. Others, like avocado, produce sensitivities triggered by latex food allergy syndrome. Sensitivity to others, like mango, can be the result of cross-reactivity due to oral allergy syndrome. We'll take a quick look at each of these types of sensitivities and at some of the fruits and vegetables that may trigger them.

Diagnosing Food Allergies

Latex food allergy syndrome (LFAS) and oral allergy syndrome (OAS) are types of cross-reactive allergies believed to occur concurrently with pollinosis, or hay fever. They're called "incomplete food allergies" to distinguish them from true, or complete, food allergies, like peanut or seafood allergies. Both are thought to be triggered by "pan-allergens," allergenic plant proteins that can produce extensive cross-reactivity in sensitive individuals.

Profilin is one such pan-allergen, occurring both in pollen and in the foods that may trigger an allergic response. It also occurs in natural rubber latex and is considered a major cause of LFAS. Recent studies have suggested that plant defensive mechanisms can organize into new groups of pan-allergens, possibly as a result of modern agricultural plant-breeding techniques, which may be one reason for the apparent increase in latex food allergies.[2]

"Complete" food allergies are caused by an immune system response that treats proteins in the offending food(s) as harmful, triggering the release of histamines and other chemicals in an effort to rid the body of the invading proteins. About 12 million people—1 of every 25 individuals—are thought to suffer from food allergies.

The most common food allergy triggers are milk, eggs, peanuts, tree nuts, fish, shellfish, soy, and wheat. Symptoms can include OAS, respiratory difficulty, hives, abdominal discomfort, nausea, vomiting, a drop in blood pressure, and, in severe cases, anaphylaxis.[3]

Incomplete food allergies are usually diagnosed like many complete food allergies, hay fever, allergic contact dermatitis, and other suspected allergies: skin prick testing or challenging with the suspected allergenic trigger. Some studies suggest that a simple clinical history taken via a validated questionnaire may be just as effective in identifying an oral allergy.[4] But challenges remain the main diagnostic tool for most types of food allergies.

Treating Food Allergies

Treatment usually involves preventing a reaction by avoiding the food in the first place. Treating the commensurate, cross-reactive pollen allergies that increase susceptibility to oral food allergies is also helpful. The Calgary Allergy Network (CAN) provides some excellent guidance for dealing with OAS.

- As soon as OAS symptoms of itching and tingling in the mouth occur, stop eating immediately. More severe reactions can occur if you don't.
- Antihistamines usually ameliorate reactions.
- Sometimes peeling a fruit or vegetable can help ameliorate reactions, as can microwaving the food briefly.
- Those who experience more severe reactions, like difficulty breathing, should consult with a doctor and always keep injectable epinephrine on hand.
- If OAS causes reactions to nuts, then all nuts, cooked or raw, should be completely avoided.

Some food allergies can also be treated through immunotherapy. A growing body of evidence suggests that gradually introducing, in a medical and monitored environment, increasing amounts of the allergenic food into the diet in some cases helps build a tolerance.[5]

But it is best to become familiar with the foods that cause problems and avoid them. This is especially true for those with predisposing conditions, like latex allergy or allergic rhinitis, which may increase the likelihood of food allergies. So let's take a closer look at some of the more common Florida food allergy triggers.

Latex Food Allergy Syndrome

Unlike complete food allergies where the allergy-triggering protein is typically resistant to heat and digestive enzymes, the proteins in LFAS and OAS are broken down by cooking and digestion. That's why many sufferers of incomplete food allergies can eat cooked foods that in their raw form trigger OAS. This is also why incomplete food allergy symptoms are mostly oral in nature, causing itching of the mouth, tongue, and throat. Despite their similarities, there are distinct differences between the two incomplete food allergy syndromes.

LFAS is most common in latex-sensitized individuals, more than half of whom show specific IgE antibodies to avocado, banana, kiwi, and potato. The most significant difference between people with LFAS and those with OAS is the severity of their allergic reactions, which can tend toward more generalized, systemic reactions in those with LFAS.[6]

Here's a look at a few common Florida fruits and vegetables that may trigger LFAS. OPALS ratings will be given where available. Many foods beyond this small sample can trigger LFAS, so consult a physician if this type of allergy is suspected, to identify possible dietary triggers.

Avocado (*Persea americana*)(3)

Avocados are evergreen trees that can grow abundantly in South Florida as a commercial crop or as a backyard fruit tree. They can

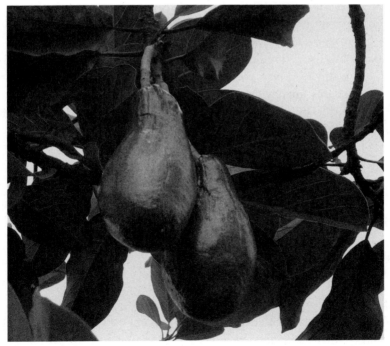

Avocado. (Photo by Dozenist. Licensed under the Creative Commons Attribution–ShareAlike 3.0 Unported license.)

reach up to 65 feet in height and produce a large green fruit around a big central pit. The avocado's flesh is buttery in color, texture, and taste and is enjoyed in a variety of ways. It can be scooped out of the shell and eaten plain or seasoned with vinegar and oil or spices. It can be mashed into a pulp for guacamole, or cut up into salads, or used as a topping or garnish for chili, stews, or sandwiches. Depending on variety, avocados contain 3–15 percent oil, making them second only to olives in their monosaturate content.[7]

Avocados have twice the potassium of bananas and are a rich source of folate, B vitamins, and other nutrients. They also contain a defense-related plant protein (Pers a 1, a class I chitinase), which produces cross-reactive allergies in those with natural rubber latex allergy, producing LFAS and sometimes OAS. In studies, the majority of those with LFAS showed strong sensitivity to avocado, with up to 53 percent in one study showing IgE-specific responses to the fruit. Although this still amounts to only about 1 percent of the general population, avocado allergy appears to be on the rise as the consumption of avocado dishes increases.[8]

Symptoms of avocado allergy are wide and varying, and can include localized mouth irritation, angioedema, urticaria, abdominal pain, asthma, nausea, vomiting, diarrhea, rhinoconjunctivitis, and, in rare cases, anaphylaxis.

Avocado oil is sometimes used in sunscreens, and reaction to sunscreens containing the oil have been documented. Excessive avocado consumption may also interfere with the anticlotting effects of warfarin.

Banana (genus *Musa*)(5)

Bananas are locally grown and imported, eaten raw as well as in a variety of ethnic dishes. They grow widely throughout Florida, although most abundantly in the southern part of the state.[9]

Despite the generally low allergenicity of bananas—it's one of the first foods babies eat, and it's commonly employed in the bland, low-fiber BRAT diet (bananas, rice, applesauce, and toast) to treat dyspepsia and gastroenteritis—about 45 percent of those with latex allergy are also allergic to bananas. Banana shares with avocado—and chestnut, passion fruit, kiwi, papaya, mango, tomato, and wheat—a class I chitinase allergen, a "defense protein" released when the plant is under stress.

Among other things, banana (and kiwi and avocado) allergy has also been found to be cross-reactive with *Ficus benjamina*. Banana can also produce food allergy symptoms in non-latex-sensitive individuals, commensurate with the increasing ripeness of the fruit. Banana allergy has several symptoms:

- Itching throat
- Gas and indigestion
- Cramps
- Diarrhea
- Vomiting
- Mouth and tongue soreness
- Canker sores
- Swollen lips
- Wheezing
- Hoarseness
- Urticaria and other rashes
- Angioedema

Perhaps because it's given to children so early in life, banana allergy can occur in infancy. Anaphylaxis has also been reported. Banana flavorings in medicines can also trigger reactions in sensitive individuals, and bananas have been known to induce migraines.[10]

Cashew Apple/Nut (*Anacardium occidentale*)

Cashew apple is a member of the Anacardium family. Besides producing the tasty cashew nut, it shares in common with its cousin poison ivy a highly allergenic, resinous latex sap containing urushiol, which can cause severe chemical contact dermatitis. The sap, which turns black on contact with air, is used in varnishes, insect repellents, and adhesives, and it occurs in the seed and fruit in complex ways that make home harvesting of the fruit in residential landscapes a hazardous venture.

Grown principally in southern frost-free areas of Florida as a landscape or botanical garden tree, cashew apple is a dense canopied evergreen that can reach 35 feet in height, although it tends more to-

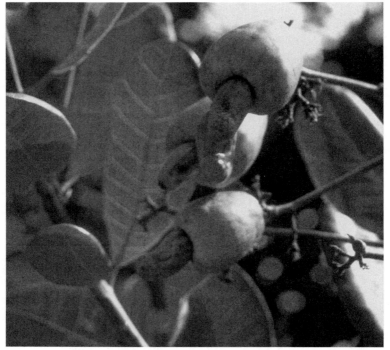

Cashew apple. (Photo by Gerard D. Hertel, West Chester University, Bugwood.org. Creative Commons Attribution 3.0 License.)

ward straggly sprawl. The pear-shaped bright red and fleshy cashew apple fruit produces the prized, cantankerous, and potentially deadly cashew nut. Home harvesting of cashew apples is discouraged for several reasons:

- The cashew nut oil is composed of poisonous phenolic lipids that can produce skin blistering.
- The sap from the cashew apple leaves, trunk, and flowers can cause dermatitis.
- Smoke from burning any part of the tree is poisonous to inhale.

Processing cashews requires professional knowledge to avoid potentially fatal reactions to improperly harvested nuts. Commercial processing is an elaborate procedure that requires immersing fruits in a hot bath to expedite shell removal and somewhat neutralize the caustic cashew nutshell liquid before the nuts are centrifuged in sawdust to further reduce toxicity.

For better or worse, the cashew nut has become ubiquitous in the American diet. It's roasted, salted, honeyed, and coated in chocolate. It's used in jams, chutneys, butters, and pesto, and it is common in Asian dishes. Perhaps not surprisingly, cashew allergy is the second most reported tree nut allergy in the United States. Sensitive individuals can also experience allergies to both the cashew nut shell oil and the nut itself. Additionally, cashew apple pollen can cause allergic rhinitis and asthma.

Cashew allergy is triggered by globulin proteins and albumins, components of the seed storage proteins in the cashew. Symptoms of cashew allergy can include atopic dermatitis, respiratory problems, and gastrointestinal distress. Oral allergy to cashews has also been reported, as has anaphylaxis. There appears to be some relationship between sensitivity to flowering cashew apple and allergy to the cashew nut.[11]

Litchi/Lychee (*Litchi chinensis*) (5)

The lychee tree is an Asian exotic prized as a broad shade tree with a large, grapelike fruit. Lychees grow best in South Florida, where the

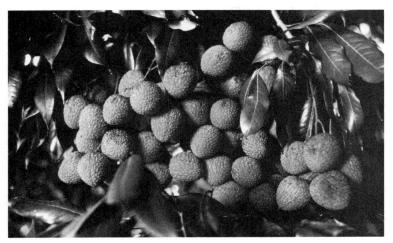

Lychee fruit. (Photo by Barry Fitzgerald, USDA Agricultural Research Service.)

fruit is eaten alone or in various recipes.[12] However, cross-reactivity with birch pollen allergy and latex allergy, as well as with apple, peach, orange, strawberry, persimmon, zucchini, and carrot, make the lychee problematic for some people. Anaphylaxis has also been reported.[13]

Mango (*Mangifera indica*) (10)

The heavenly sweet mango, a regional and ethnic favorite throughout Florida that makes its way into salads, chutneys, beverages, jellies, and ice cream, is also, unfortunately, a member of the Anacharidae family of highly allergenic plants. It is closely related to the cashew and triggers allergies via everything from its pollen to its sap. In something akin to adding insult to injury, overexposure to poison oak or poison ivy can produce cross-reactions upon consumption of mango.[14]

A beautiful tree with leathery dark green leaves, there are literally thousands of varieties of mango, and it grows abundantly in South Florida backyards and commercial groves. Ripe fruits have a lovely blush, and when stripped of their thick, leathery peel, they offer a sweet, juicy, messy treat rich in phosphorous, potassium, and other vitamins and minerals.[15]

It can also offer up LFAS, OAS, and contact dermatitis. Thanks to class I chitinases, it is highly cross-reactive with birch pollen for 10–15 percent of those suffering from birch allergy, as well as cross-reactive with celery and carrot. The leaves, stems, and fruit contain, among other things, urushiol and limonene, the problematic components of contact allergy plants like poison ivy. Mango tree pollen can also cause allergic rhinitis and asthma, and anaphylaxis has occurred.[16]

Papaya (*Carica papaya*) (1)

Papaya grows throughout much of Florida and is used in a variety of dishes, eaten fresh by itself, ripe or green, and employed in salads, drinks, or desserts. Rich in vitamins and nutrients, it is popular dried, candied, and processed into jams and preserves.[17]

The female papaya plants are pollen-free and considered a good

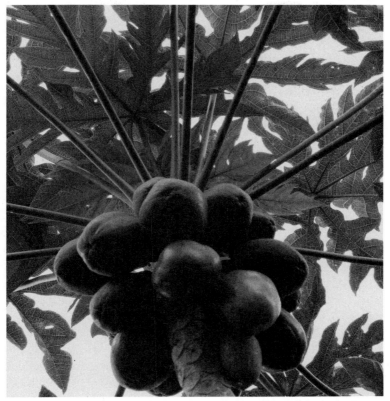

Papaya fruit. (Photo by Forest and Kim Starr, U.S. Geological Survey, Bugwood.org. Creative Commons Attribution 3.0 License.)

landscape plant for those with pollen allergies. But the fruit contains the problematic class I chitinase, which triggers LFAS, with latex present in both the fruit and the plant itself, as well as complete food allergies that can cause urticaria, colitis, and even anaphylaxis. The papain in papaya can also trigger OAS, as well as sneezing, rhinitis, and gastrointestinal symptoms.[18]

Passion Fruit (family Passifloraceae)(3)

An ordinary-looking vine with an extraordinary flower, the passion vine is full of contradictions. Also known as the maypop, presum-

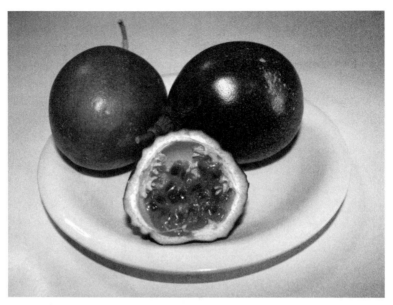

Passion fruit. (Photo by Suguri F. Permission is granted to copy, distribute and/or modify this document under the terms of the GNU Free Documentation License, version 1.2 or any later version.)

ably for the popping sound the fruit makes when crushed, which served as sport for pioneer children, a few varieties of passion flower grow wild throughout Florida.

The plant gets its common name from the religious connotations evoked by its complex form, like the Star of Bethlehem seemingly apparent in the half-opened flower, and the 30 pieces of silver for which Judas sold Jesus in the appropriately numbered round spots beneath the leaves. Numerous other associations are made with respect to the anthers, stigma, and feathery tendrils around the petals.

Most people know the passion vine for its pretty fence line flowers or as an attractive trellis plant. But the fruit is also popular, cooked or raw. It can be processed into jams, syrups, and drinks, and the leaves have long been used in teas and tonics, most often for their sedative or calming properties.[19]

However, some of those same sedative-evoking chemical compounds, which include alkaloids, terpenes, and cyanogenic glyco-

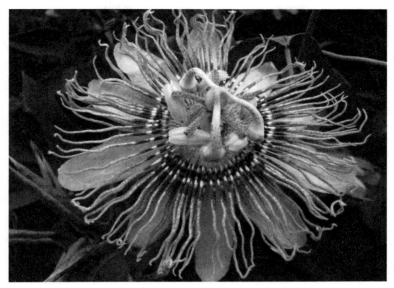

Passion flower. (Photo by Rebekah D. Wallace, Bugwood.org. Creative Commons Attribution 3.0 License.)

sides, can also be allergenic or toxic.[20] Passion fruit can trigger latex food allergy in sensitive individuals due to a class I chitinase protein that can produce cross-reactivity with kiwi, papaya, mango, tomato, and wheat as well.

In children, cross-reactivity with passion fruit may also extend to apricot, banana, cherry, grape, peach, and pineapple.[21] Consequently, anyone with latex allergy should take precautions with the use of fresh passion fruit or herbal preparations using the fruit or leaves.

Pineapple (*Ananas comosus*) (2)

Pineapple is common in regional and ethnic dishes in Florida, and while not a commercial crop here, it is available in grocery stores and easily propagated in the home garden. The pineapple plant is a bromeliad, and the pineapple fruit is actually a "syncarp," the fusion of the fruits of many individual flowers into one single fruit. Other syncarps include magnolia and raspberry.

Allergy to pineapple is common, expressing itself as latex food allergy, through cross-reactivity to rye grass pollen and with papain, and as a complete food allergy, capable of producing asthma, rhinitis, and gastrointestinal symptoms. Pineapple is reported to be one of the most common triggers of atopic dermatitis.[22]

Oral Allergy Syndrome

As a child, one of our daughters would always complain about her mouth and throat itching when she ate raw carrots. She didn't seem to have any other symptoms or to be experiencing any seasonal allergies. She never had a problem eating cooked carrots. When she was much older and tried raw carrots again, she no longer experienced the problem.

It wasn't until relatively recently that we figured out she had been experiencing OAS. Typically, oral allergy syndrome, also known as "pollen-food allergy syndrome," is caused only by a raw fruit or vegetable to which sensitivity is triggered by a concurrent pollen allergy. Foods that produce OAS can often be eaten when cooked or processed. OAS is usually mild, as was the case for our daughter, causing an itching or tingling sensation in the mouth when eating an offending food, although more extensive reactions may include swelling of the mouth, face, tongue, and throat.[23]

The AAAAI estimates that about a third of people with allergies can develop OAS. While symptoms may worsen during a particular pollen season, OAS can occur at any time of year. It is usually diagnosed by a positive test for a specific food or pollen, along with a history of oral symptoms. Sensitive individuals don't need to avoid all the foods that can cause OAS, but only those to which they've experienced a reaction.

OAS-causing foods may vary by pollen trigger.[24] Allergy to birch pollen produces the most symptoms, including reactions to plants in the apple family, which also includes pears; the plum family, including almonds, apricots, cherry, nectarine, peach, and prune; the parsley family, which includes carrots, celery, fennel, and parsnip; and walnuts.

Ragweed pollen allergy can trigger oral allergy reactions to bananas and melons. Mugwort can produce reactions to carrots and celery as well as apples, melons and watermelons. And grass pollen allergy can produce OAS to melons, kiwis, oranges, tomatoes, potatoes, and peanuts.

Many of the foods that commonly cause OAS can be found not only in Florida grocery stores but also in backyards across the state—things like avocado, mango, citrus, and homegrown herbs. Of those, citrus is one of the most common backyard crops in Florida and deserves a closer look.

Citrus (4–5)

Fragrant when flowering, varied but usually attractive in appearance, citrus is practically synonymous with Florida. Its cultivation history here dates to the mid-1500s, when Spanish explorers planted the first orange trees near St. Augustine. A wide variety of citrus can be found growing throughout the state, commercially in about 576,000 acres of citrus groves containing more than 75 million citrus trees, as well as in backyards from the Keys to Jacksonville. Florida produces more than 70 percent of the nation's citrus and is the world's leading producer of grapefruit.[25]

The most commonly grown citrus in Florida are oranges, grapefruit, tangerines, tangelos, lemons, and limes. Allergies to all types of citrus can occur as complete allergies or as a result of cross-reactivity to allergies to grass or tree pollens. Grapefruit, oranges, and tangelos (a hybrid of the two) are all cross-reactive with one another and with allergies to grass and other tree pollens, and they can produce allergic symptoms ranging from atopic dermatitis to OAS.[26]

Ten to 15 percent of those with birch pollen allergy are cross-reactive to several fruits, including oranges. The main allergic components in oranges have actually been found to reside in the fruit's seeds, rather than in the pulp or juice.[27] But the seeds can be difficult to avoid and easily become mixed with pressed juices and in other preparations. Orange allergy can also occur as a complete food allergy.

Complete Food Allergies

Since there are plenty of literary, scholastic, and medical resources to address food allergies today, we'll just look briefly here at some Florida-specific food allergies.

Citrus: Oranges and Limes

In addition to OAS, oranges can also trigger complete food allergies and are considered one of the top ten food allergens affecting children ages 7 to 10.[28] Symptoms of orange allergy include nausea, pruritis (sensation of itching), gastrointestinal distress, rhinitis, low blood pressure, and, in extreme cases, anaphylaxis. Oranges are also a common cause of migraine headaches and may produce phyto-photodermatitis.

Two types of limes are typically grown in Florida: key limes and Tahiti limes. Key limes are tiny and popular in the pie of the same name. Tahiti limes are larger. Phytophotodermatitis is the most common allergic reaction to limes, but as members of the citrus family, they can also produce food allergy symptoms.

Carambola (*Averrhoa carambola L*)(1)

Carambola, also known as "star fruit," is a medium-sized, usually evergreen tree (it can be deciduous in cooler climates), growing to around 30 feet tall. It produces a waxy, yellow four- to five-celled fruit that when sliced creates a characteristic star-shaped section of fruit that is crisp, juicy, and varying in sweetness. Introduced from Southeast Asia a century ago, the fruit is now grown commercially throughout South Florida. It is used in fruit salads, sauces, wines, and jellies.[29]

Carambola fruit is high in potassium, and very ripe carambola fruit is also high in oxalic acid, making it potentially unsafe for those with kidney disease. Conversely, the fruit has traditionally been used to treat hemorrhaging, fevers, eczema, and other ills, and for the home economist, it has a reputation as a stain remover and metal cleaner and polish.

While allergy to carambola is rare among healthy individuals, and cross-reaction with other allergens hasn't been reported, there

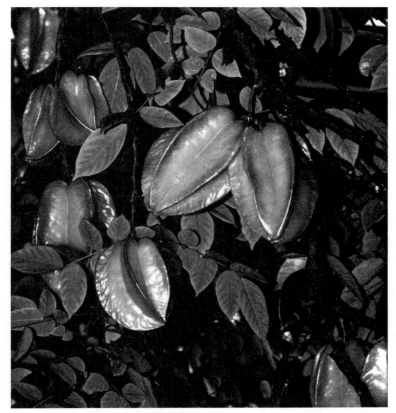

Carambola fruit. (Photo by Scott Bauer, USDA Agricultural Research Service.)

appear to be enough cases of hypersensitivity to the fruit by people with impaired renal function to at least mention it.[30] Sometimes known as "star fruit intoxication,"[31] uremic patients, or those on some sort of dialytic treatment, have developed hiccups, confusion, nausea, vomiting, and even seizures, with occasionally fatal consequences.

Coconut (*Cocos nucifera*)

Coconut palms grow along the warmer tropical coastal regions of South Florida as a picturesque ornamental whose large nut is popular in regional and ethnic dishes. Coconut is also a component of various cosmetics, soaps, cooking oil, and margarine.[32] Crowned by an elegant spray of fronds, coconut palms can reach 100 feet in height. The nut of the coconut palm can be more than 15 inches long and a foot wide.

As a child, I remember watching my Cuban relatives expertly husk and then, with a swift machete stroke, cleave off the top of a big green coconut for us to drink the sweet "milk" and then parcel out the coconut "meat," the pure white flesh lining the inside of the nut. We routinely played with coconuts, kicking them, tossing them, and decorating them. (Who hasn't seen coconuts carved into monkeys and other shapes in Florida souvenir shops?)

For some people, though, the coconut, which is immunologically similar to soy, produces allergy symptoms. Cross-reactivity is the most common trigger of coconut allergy, especially in those allergic to walnuts and hazelnuts. While contact dermatitis is the most common reaction, since coconut oil is found in a large number of products, it can also produce OAS, and there are some reports of latex-related allergy to coconut. Some individuals are also sensitive to the pollen produced by the coconut palm.[33]

Food allergy reactions, however, are IgE mediated, sometimes on the level of peanut or other tree nut allergies. Coconut food allergy symptoms can include oral itching, abdominal pain or discomfort, facial swelling, coughing, wheezing, and respiratory problems. As with many food allergies, reactions can be delayed from four to six hours, and anaphylaxis has been reported.

Guava (genus *Psidium*) (3)

Another delicious local delicacy, guava fruit ranges broadly in flavor and aroma and comes in dozens of varieties, although two basic types—pink, or red pulp, and white pulp fruit bearers—are usually grown in Florida. Closely related to rose-apple and clove, guava can be eaten fresh, added as a garnish or flavoring in desserts, processed into pastes, cooked in pies, or served as a juice.[34] As a child, one of my favorite after-school treats was a plate of jellied guava and cream cheese on Cuban crackers.

For some people, however, guava can produce symptoms similar to that experienced in people sensitive to peaches, bananas, manda-

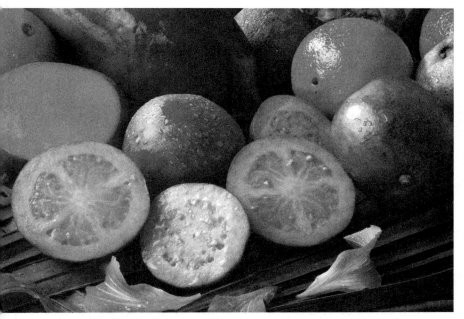

Guava fruit. The juicy sliced fruit in the center, which is bright pink in color, is high in antioxidants. (Photo by Penny Greb, USDA Agricultural Research Service.)

rin oranges, and strawberries.[35] Symptoms can include rhinitis and itching of the throat.

Mango

The delicious mango, unfortunately, crops up again in the complete food allergy category as well as in LFAS and OAS discussions. Although mango allergy is more often due to latex allergy, it can also produce outright food allergy in sensitive individuals. Tampa resident Jodi Baudean was excited to try mango when she first moved to Florida years ago.

"After living here a few years, it just seemed like mango was everywhere. I finally asked at the local market and had them help me pick out a ripe mango. I brought it home, cut it open, and tasted it. It was wonderful, maybe the best fruit I had ever tasted," she recalled.

"The flesh was tender like a ripe peach, but the flavor was so much more delicious. Then the inside of my cheeks began to swell and then my throat. I have never tasted it again."

She's not alone. Mango is among the top five foods implicated in anaphylactic reactions, after celery, shellfish, fish, and peanuts.

Strawberry (family Rosaceae)

While not an indigenous plant, strawberries are a big crop in Florida, with Hillsborough County alone producing about 15 percent of the nation's strawberries and almost all of the strawberries grown nationwide during the winter. Strawberries are grown on over 8,000 acres, with an economic impact of $272 million annually.[36] Floridians in Central Florida celebrate the fruit at the Plant City Strawberry Festival every February, and "U-pic" strawberry orchards are abundant.

Eaten raw, alone, or in salads, used as a garnish, pureed into smoothies, cooked into pies and cakes, and used in ice cream, strawberries are a perennial and inexpensive favorite here. They're also a common allergenic food for many people, triggering allergies through cross-reactivity with birch pollen or with other fruits like pears and peaches. Strawberries can trigger OAS as well as complete food allergies. Allergy symptoms can include gastrointestinal distress, atopic dermatitis, asthma, and rhinitis.[37]

In Summary

- Dietary allergies to common Florida fruits, vegetables, and nuts can take any combination of three basic forms: latex food allergy syndrome (LFAS), oral allergy syndrome (OAS), and complete food allergies.
- LFAS and OAS are incomplete food allergies: cross-reactive allergies believed to be concurrent with pollinosis (hay fever).
- Proteins involved in incomplete food allergies can typically be broken down by heat, so OAS and LFAS sufferers can often eat cooked foods that eaten raw would trigger oral symptoms.
- LFAS is most common in latex-sensitized individuals, more than half of whom show specific IgE antibodies to latex-con-

taining fruits and vegetables like avocado, banana, cashew, papaya, and pineapple.

- OAS is caused by the ingestion of a raw fruit or vegetable to which sensitivity is triggered by a concurrent pollen allergy.
- OAS symptoms, usually mild, include itching or tingling sensations in the mouth in response to a stimulus food. More serious OAS reactions include swelling of the mouth, face, tongue, and throat.
- Peeling or briefly microwaving foods to which one experiences OAS can reduce or eliminate reactions.
- Foods to which OAS may develop vary by pollen trigger. Allergy to birch pollen, for example, produces most of the OAS symptoms, including reactions to plants in the apple, plum, parsley and walnut families.
- The most common food allergy triggers are milk, eggs, peanuts, tree nuts, fish, shellfish, soy, and wheat, although food allergies to commonly grown Florida foods like oranges, mango, carambola, coconut, guava, and strawberries also exist.
- Food allergy symptoms can include OAS, respiratory difficulty, hives, abdominal discomfort, nausea, vomiting, drop in blood pressure and, in severe cases, anaphylaxis.
- Food allergies are typically diagnosed by skin prick testing or challenging with the suspected food trigger.
- Immunotherapy is the most common food allergy treatment, but avoidance is the best solution.

Part IV

The Life Aquatic

How inappropriate to call this planet Earth when it is quite clearly
Ocean.

Arthur C. Clarke

BeachHunter.net provides an obscure and wonderful free e-booklet
bearing the long and possibly unsettling title *How to Be Safe from
Sharks, Jellyfish, Stingrays, Rip Currents, and Other Scary Things on Florida Beaches and Coastal Waters.*[1] Written by David McRee, the table of
contents reads like the Little Shop of Seaside Horrors.

Ten pages of the booklet are devoted to sharks and shark bite
information. Twenty pages examine drown-proofing, rip currents,
and heavy surf. Twenty-five pages or so cover things that bite, sting,
pinch, or stab, including birds with sharp bills, and several dozen
pages look at water quality, bad weather, the sun, fish, shellfish poisoning, and even "holes on the beach." The Life Aquatic in Florida can
definitely pose some hazards!

The fact is, though, that an educated Florida beachgoer is a safer
Florida beachgoer. As beautiful as our shores and surf are, they are
first and foremost habitat for thousands of species of sea life, many

of which protect themselves in ways that humans find uncomfortable and occasionally deadly. There's no shortage of things along the beach or in the water that can cause injuries, including allergies and contact irritants.

Jellyfish stings and punctures from sea urchins and various bony fish can produce serious allergic reactions. Bacteria and algae in the water at certain times of year can trigger extensive itching, conjunctivitis, and hoarseness. Certain corals and anemones can cause the equivalent of chemical burns on contact. And seafood can produce respiratory allergies as deadly as anaphylaxis. But before we explore some of these threats more closely, and before you swear off the beach altogether, a little perspective might be helpful.

First, as with everything else we've looked at in the preceding chapters, a little knowledge goes a long way toward keeping beachgoers and recreational water enthusiasts safe and healthy. And second, many of the allergies and irritants we'll look at in this section are, for most people, statistically unlikely to cause serious harm, especially considering the sheer number of people flirting with more ordinary and far more likely disasters on our waterways each year. For perspective, consider the following:

- Nearly 80 percent of Florida's population—over 12 million people—reside in 35 coastal counties.
- They share more than 825 miles of sandy beaches with millions of visitors. Honeymoon Island alone, in Dunedin on the Gulf Coast, hosts over a million visitors annually. Other top-rated seaside parks like St. Andrews in Panama City Beach, Bill Baggs Cape Florida State Park in Key Biscayne, Gasparilla Island State Park in Boca Grande, and Sebastian Inlet State Park in Melbourne Beach, each draw 700,000 to nearly a million visitors annually.[2]

- Marine biodiversity in Florida is immense, with the Florida Straits containing nearly 700 species of marine life in one concentrated region.[3]
- The Indian River Lagoon supports more than 3,000 species of estuarine plants and animals, comprising perhaps one of the most diverse marine environments in the continental United States.[4]

Millions of people, and millions of sea creatures, all vying for a few hundred feet of shoreline, and yet the greatest cause of water-related fatality in Florida—400 people annually—is drowning.[5] Hundreds more are injured in boating accidents each year.[6] Both of these dangers are self-inflicted and usually preventable.

And so, too, are the rare encounters with the various and sundry creatures that typically seek only to avoid being stepped upon or eaten. In this section, we'll look at ways to enjoy our remarkable seashores, lakes, and rivers without becoming victims of our own ignorance. We'll get (safely) up close and personal with

- Cnidaria, the family of stinging sea life that includes jellyfish, sea anemones, corals, and the Portuguese man-of-war;
- bony fish and echinoderms (sea urchins and sea cucumbers);
- water-borne allergens that produce things like red tide and hot tub rash; and
- seafood and shellfish allergies

So put on your wading shoes and do the stingray shuffle. We're going into the water!

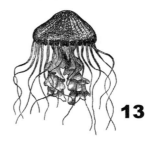

13

The Sting of Cnidaria

Most of us, I suppose, are a little nervous of the sea.
No matter what its smiles may be, we doubt its friendship.

H. M. Tomlinson

The phylum Cnidaria (pronounced with a silent *c*) is an ancient and diverse group of aquatic creatures over 11,000 species strong. There are four major groups of Cnidarian: [1]

1. Anthozoa—true corals, anemones, and sea pens
2. Cubozoa—including the highly toxic box jellies
3. Hydrozoa—including hydroids, fire corals, and the Portuguese man-of-war
4. Scyphozoa—the true jellyfish

Cnidaria have some amazing biological adaptations. They have two distinct body forms—the stationary polyp, like anemones, and the free swimming medusa, like jellyfish. Their bodies are composed of two layers of tissue that include nerves and muscles. And they have a single orifice that serves as both mouth and anus and is surrounded by nematocysts, or stinging tentacles.

Notably, the word *Cnidaria* stems from the Greek *cnidos,* which means "stinging nettle." The nematocysts, which vary in length by species, are venom-filled hollow tubes lined with tiny spines that aid in penetration and venom delivery. Venom release is triggered either by physical contact or chemical stimulation. The venom, which can be injected at the rate of 2 meters per second—up to 2–5 psi in something like a man-of-war—is a cocktail of proteins, carbohydrates, and other components that are efficiently distributed throughout the body by increased heart rates when a victim reacts in fear or flight.[2]

As Cnidaria can't distinguish between a hungry fish and a blundering bather, they respond with indiscriminate inflictions of varying degrees of pain and, in rare but reported cases, commensurate allergic reactions to the protein component in the venom. While reactions may be rare, Cnidaria are responsible for more envenomation reports than any other marine animal.[3] Up to 200,000 jellyfish stings are reported in Florida each year.[4]

But let's take an alphabetical look and start with Anthozoa, the class of Cnidaria where the stinging sea anemones can be found.

Anthozoa

The Anthozoa have three forms:

- True "stony" corals that form the foundation of big and beautiful reefs so enjoyed by Florida divers
- Sea pens and sea pansies, as harmless as they sound
- Sea anemones, beautiful but toxic flowery sea creatures

Although members of this class may look like plants, they are all carnivorous animals. The only Anthozoa of toxicological interest here are the sea anemones. Anemones vary in size, coloration, and elaborateness.

Dozens of species live in Florida waters, but all are essentially the same. Anemones have a tubular body that terminates in a suction cup–like base, which it attaches to coral or other hard surfaces, and a slitlike mouth at the top, surrounded by stinging tentacles. With their tentacles swaying gently in the current, anemones lie in wait for prey to be drawn into their nematocysts, which effectively paralyze small fish and crustaceans so that the anemones can consume them.

Obviously, sea anemones aren't something most people will encounter. But divers or snorkelers poking about with unprotected hands or brushing a bare limb past an anemone are likely to get

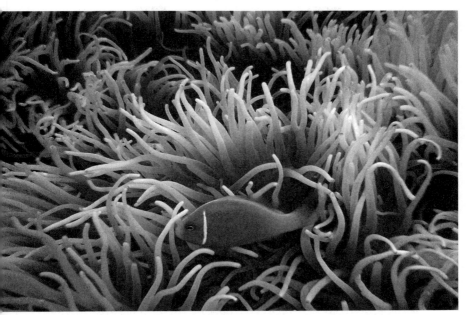

Sea anemone. (Photo by David Burdick, courtesy of National Oceanic and Atmospheric Administration, U.S. Department of Commerce [NOAA/ USDC].)

stung. In Florida, sponge divers may also develop "sponge fisherman's disease" from frequent contact with anemones that live within the sponges they harvest. But the most commonly encountered anemone is the bulb or bubble tip anemone. Stings are usually mild, but on rare occasion they have produced reactions as severe as liver failure.[5]

Ordinarily, though, an anemone sting may, at most, cause a purplish mark, rashes, and inflammation at the site of the sting. At least anemones are fairly well anchored—victims have to go to them to get stung. Jellyfish are another story.

Jellyfish

While several amorphous, floating jellylike sea creatures are colloquially called jellyfish, there are distinguishing differences between species. We'll look at the box jellyfish and the "true" jellyfish together here because, regardless of which one stings you, reactions and treatments are similar.

In recent years, jellyfish "blooms" have resulted in beach hazards and injuries throughout Florida. Although jellyfish reside in Florida waters year-round, they are most abundant in the summer, which is also when beachgoers are most abundant. And, unfortunately, what's bad for nature in many respects—things like climate change and poor water quality, which are factors in the decline of some Cnidaria species, especially corals—may create favorable conditions for jellyfish.

In August 2007, 300 people were stung by jellyfish on a single day at New Smyrna Beach.[6] None of the injuries produced severe reactions. But jellyfish are among the most dangerous creatures in the sea.

Cubozoa

The Cubozoa class of Cnidaria includes two of the most toxic marine creatures in the world: the box jellyfish and sea wasp. Box jellyfish are most common in Australian waters, where they are known to have killed 70 people. There are small varieties of box jellyfish in Florida, but none apparently as dangerous as the Australian varieties, although a new species, the Bonaire banded box jellyfish, was discovered in the Caribbean in 2001 and is still under study.[7]

There have also been reports of an anaphylactic response to box jelly stings in Florida, called Irukandji syndrome.[8] Originally identified in Australia, Irukandji syndrome is characterized by a delayed response (half an hour to two hours following an initial sting) that includes severe low back pain, abdominal cramps, nausea, vomiting, profuse sweating, headache, agitation, tachycardia, and hypertension. Symptoms may progress to pulmonary edema and cardiac arrest.[9] So far, though, serious reactions to box jellyfish stings in Florida are mostly anecdotal.

The sea wasp is another story. Sometimes the names sea wasp and box jellyfish are used interchangeably, but they're two different creatures. Sea wasps are generally larger than box jellyfish, up to 4½ inches long, and nocturnal, coming into shallow water at night to

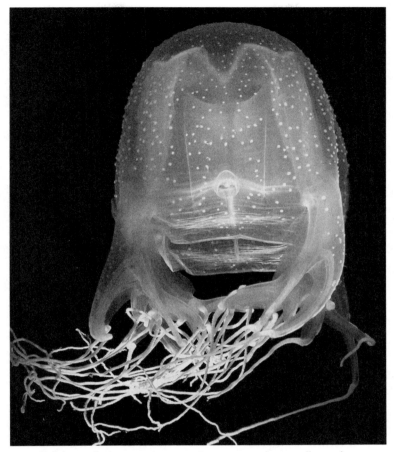

Box jellyfish, similar in appearance to the sea wasp, but smaller and a daytime feeder. (Photo by Bastian Bentlage, Northeast Fisheries Science Center's National Systematics Laboratory, courtesy of NOAA/USDC.)

feed near shore.[10] Until recently, the sea wasp wasn't thought to live in Florida. But in 2002, a swarm sent hundreds of beachgoers to emergency rooms along the east coast of the state. While there were no serious injuries in that case, sea wasp stings are extremely painful, can produce long-lasting inflamed eruptions on the skin, and are potentially deadly.[11] Now known to occur along the Gulf of Mexico, in the Caribbean, and along the Atlantic coast, sea wasps have killed 15–20 percent of their victims, especially children.[12]

Scyphozoa

The Scyphozoa class of Cnidaria contains the "true" jellyfish.[13] Those most commonly encountered in Florida are sea nettles, lion's mane, cannonball, upside-down, moon, and thimble jellyfish.

Sea nettles, the textbook perfect jellyfish with the classic bell shape and long dangling tentacles, swarm in large numbers, triggering hazard flags along beaches statewide. Their sting can be painful and may produce redness, swelling, and a rash. Allergic reactions can include respiratory distress, muscle cramps, and a feeling of chest constriction.[14]

Lion's mane jellyfish are the largest species. Most common in colder Arctic waters, where they can grow to be 7 feet across with tentacles 120 feet long, lion's mane jellyfish can occur in Atlantic waters but are fairly easy to avoid and rarely cause problems in Florida.

Upside-down jellyfish, as their name implies, swim upside-down and often anchor themselves on the floor of mangrove beds and other shallow bay and estuary areas, resembling seagrass. Also known as Cassiopeia, these jellyfish cloaked sea beds throughout Southwest Florida in 2007. The unusually large bloom was thought to be caused by drought and high levels of nutrients in the water that triggered algae blooms on which the jellyfish feed.[15]

Since the jellyfish reside upside-down on the sea floor, just swimming over them can expose swimmers to the stinging cells released in mucosal material by the jellyfish. The resulting stings are mild but extremely itchy.[16]

The cannonball jellyfish is a common Florida jelly with a large compact bell and short, frilly tentacles. It's a strong swimmer, and although abundant, occurring in the millions throughout the northern Gulf of Mexico and along the Atlantic coast, it rarely stings people. People, on the other hand, sometimes enjoy eating cannonball jellyfish, which are one of the state's commercial seafood harvests. The cannonball has a dense body and is high in collagen.[17]

Moon jellyfish are often found washed up on beaches after a storm, with their horseshoe-shaped gonads visible through their clear bells. Moon jellies are a favorite sea turtle snack and a regular companion of local divers, who often report diving through "walls"

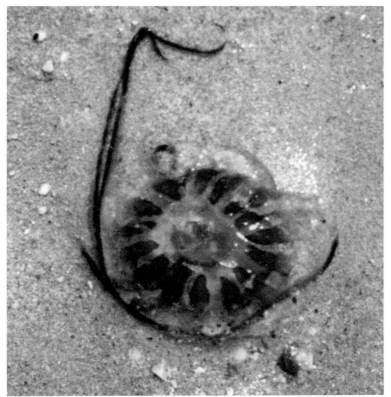

Sea nettle on beach. (Photo by Mary Hollinger, NESDIS/NODC biologist, courtesy of NOAA/USDC.)

of moon jellyfish. Like all jellyfish, they sting, although reactions are generally milder than those attributed to other types of jellyfish, producing localized itching, pain, swelling, and redness.[18]

Thimble jellyfish are responsible for an allergic reaction of another kind: seabather's eruption, an itchy rash that made its medical debut in 1949, right here in Florida. Clinically described as pruritic papular eruption, the condition is caused by the tiny thimble jellyfish's infinitesimal larvae, which are common in shallow waters, especially in the Martin County area in Florida.[19] Sometimes erroneously referred to as "sea lice," the thimble jellyfish larvae and some species of sea anemone become trapped in great abundance in swim-

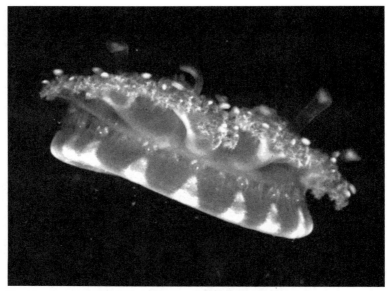

Upside-down jellyfish. (Photo courtesy of NOAA/USDC.)

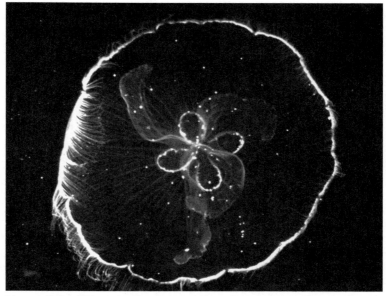

Moon jellyfish. (Photo by Florida Keys National Marine Sanctuary Staff, courtesy of NOAA/USDC.)

wear, where they sting copiously and produce severe itching that can last up to ten days, with or without any outward skin eruptions or rashes.[20]

The itching and rashes that may appear are due to an allergic reaction to the proteins in the larval Cnidaria toxins. The reactions typically occur upon leaving the water, when swimwear drains, trapping the larvae under increasing pressure between bathing suit and skin and triggering nematocysts to discharge. Staying in swimwear for a long time, showering in freshwater, or rubbing with a towel can worsen reactions.

To add insult to itchy injury, irritation can recur days or even weeks later, long after infected swimwear, clothing, and towels have been laundered, since nematocyst cells are mechanical in nature and can continue to "fire" even after the living creature they're normally attached to dies or is removed.[21] This is why beachcombers are cautioned against touching dead jellyfish along the shore.

Hydrozoa

The Hydrozoa class of Cnidarians is where you find the communal dwelling corals, including fire coral and the Portuguese man-of-war. It's easy to forget that corals are animals. Coral reefs are actually networked communities of Hydrozoa that got their start by attaching themselves to some hard substrate from which they continued to "bud." For our purposes, the main difference between the two species we're looking at here, fire coral and the Portuguese man-of-war, is that one is anchored and the other is free-floating.

Fire coral, for all intents and purposes, won't be an issue for most people. But if you're a diver or snorkeler, it helps to be aware of the hazards it poses. Two basic species of fire coral can be found in Florida waters: branching fire coral, which is bright to light creamy yellow, typically with smooth, cylindrical branches, and blade fire coral, which is brown to light creamy yellow, growing in fan-shaped, uneven blades.[22]

Fire coral has the unfortunate ability to seem dead while being very much alive and able to inflict injury via whiplike stinging cells.[23] Contact with floating nematocysts from these corals can cause severe burning sensations.

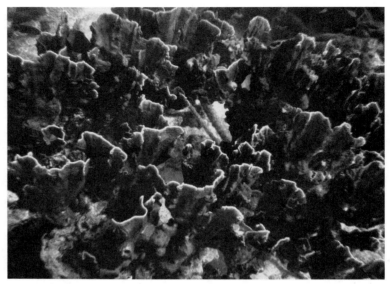

Fire coral. (Photo courtesy of "Bonaire 2008: Exploring Coral Reef Sustainability with New Technologies," Office of Ocean Exploration and Research, NOAA/USDC.)

Box fire coral, appearing much as its name suggests, is less common than branching and blade fire corals, occurring sporadically throughout the Caribbean. While contact may produce a stinging sensation, unlike the other two fire corals, box fire coral isn't considered toxic.[24]

Most encounters are the result of swimmers or divers accidentally bumping into the coral or swimming near or above it and being exposed to its mucosal release of stinging nematocyst cells. This invariably produces a severe burning sensation on contact and sometimes causes inflammation, welts, and regional lymphatic swelling. As with seabather's eruption and most jellyfish encounters, the impulse to wash the affected area with freshwater only worsens it, triggering unfired nematocysts that may remain on the skin to release their toxins.[25]

While it may seem odd to group fire coral and the Portuguese man-of-war together, the man-of-war is more akin to coral than to jellyfish. This remarkable creature is actually a colony of four separate unisexual organisms:

- The pneumatophore—the characteristic gas-filled purple sail or float
- Dactylozooids, the tentacles, which contain cnidocytes, or stinging cells
- Gastrozooids, or feeding polyps
- Gonozooids, which produce gametes for reproduction[26]

Unlike jellyfish, whose locomotion results from a combination of pulsations and undulations, the man-of-war is at the mercy of wind and currents, driven across the ocean much like the ship for which it is named. The pneumatophore sail is filled with air containing a large concentration of carbon monoxide, which the man-of-war can regulate to adjust the depth at which it floats. It feeds by making a great stinging net of its bluish tentacles, which can reach 150 feet in length.[27]

I have personal experience with the extent of their tentacled reach, having once attempted to give a man-of-war what I thought was a sufficiently wide berth as I waded along a sandbar in Miami. With the little blue sail a good 20 yards away at least, I was surprised to suddenly feel a burning sensation along my legs. I hightailed it out of the water, flailing as I went and causing quite a few other people to flail preemptively out of the way as well. I was met on shore by an indulgent lifeguard ready with a soothing vinegar solution and calamine lotion.

The pain and burning soon eased, and by the end of the day, I'd almost forgotten about the encounter. It actually hadn't stung me as extensively as I'd feared. But a week later, I experienced intense itching where I'd been stung, which continued to occur off and on for a few more days. I've studiously avoided man-of-wars in the water and on the beach ever since.

Sting encounters can leave long, linear red streaks—tentacle prints —and produce intense pain. Allergic responses range from the itching I experienced, which can be ameliorated with antihistamines, to cardiac and respiratory problems and in some cases anaphylactic shock.

Allergic Reactions to Cnidaria

Most people will never have a severe allergic reaction to the stings from sea anemones, jellyfish, fire corals, or the Portuguese man-

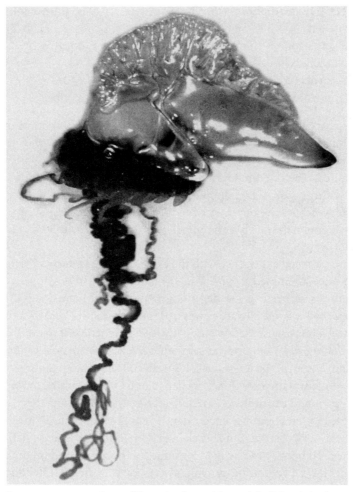

Portuguese man-of-war. (Photo by Bruce Moravchik, "Islands in the Stream Expedition 2002," Office of Ocean Exploration and Research, courtesy of NOAA/USDC.)

of-war. While common, most stings will never present as anything more than temporarily painful welts and swelling and maybe some commensurate itching for a few hours or days.[28]

A small number of people will experience more severe reactions like papules (bumps), vesicles (blisters), and skin necrosis (the death of skin cells). Sometimes hyperpigmentation (skin color changes) can occur, as happened to half of those afflicted in the 2002 sea wasp invasion, many of whom have permanent hyperpigmentation.[29]

Other signs of severe allergic reaction that require immediate medical attention may include low blood pressure, headache, nausea, vomiting, diarrhea, muscle spasms, fever, tightening of the chest or throat, swelling of the tongue and lips, and respiratory distress.[30] If nematocysts affect the eyes, conjunctivitis, corneal ulcerations, and eyelid edema can result.[31] Most severe reactions will occur within 15 to 30 minutes of a sting and usually no more than six hours afterwards.

The first symptom of seabather's eruption is a tingling sensation inside swimwear, often while the bather is still in the water and usually (and unfortunately) along breasts and groin areas and within the cuffs of wetsuits. Rashes of dense red bumps develop within a few hours of swimming, accompanied by severe itching, which can last for several weeks. About a fifth of patients also report feeling generally unwell, with fevers and fatigue. Children may develop stomach upset.[32]

Treating Cnidaria Stings

Treatment for almost all Cnidaria encounters is about the same.[33]

- Neutralize the sting with vinegar (most effective), 50-percent-diluted household ammonia, or papain for at least 30 minutes. A product called Smithwick's StingMate, containing a 5 percent acetic acid solution similar to vinegar, has also shown promise in treating jellyfish stings.[34]
- Remove any visible nematocysts in the skin. This is accomplished most effectively with shaving cream and a razor while rinsing the razor after each pass. Nematocysts can also be removed by applying talcum powder to vinegar-moistened skin to create a layer of damp powder that can then be gently scraped away with a wooden tongue depressor or the edge of a card, taking nematocysts with it.

- Use hot packs or soak in warm saltwater to help break down Cnidaria toxins. Avoid rinsing with freshwater, which can activate nematocysts!
- Apply topical corticosteroids or take antihistamines.

With seabather's eruption, it's important to remember that stinging cells may remain in swimwear even after washing and drying, so several washings may be in order. Rinsing swimwear in alcohol or vinegar first may help neutralize and remove nematocysts more effectively.

Protecting against Cnidaria Encounters

A good offense is the best defense, and short of staying out of the water altogether, dive suits have long provided the best protection against jellyfish and other hazards. More practical for the garden variety beachgoer, however, is Safe Sea, a sunblock with jellyfish protection made by Nidaria Technology. The sunblock, when applied prior to entering the water, purports to act as a "sting inhibitor," blocking nematocyst discharge. Early reports on its effectiveness are promising.[35]

Here are some more protective measures:

- Wear water shoes! These tough, comfortable mesh shoes do a great job of protecting feet while wading.
- Don't touch things that can't be identified.
- Wear dive gloves.
- Get out of the water when warned to do so or on spotting jellyfish. A purple flag flying at beaches or lifeguard stations indicates hazardous marine life.
- Don't dangle arms and legs over the side of a boat, especially while chumming, and especially at dusk or at night.
- Avoid floating seaweed, which harbors the tiny larvae that cause seabather's eruption.
- Remove swimwear promptly after swimming, especially after possible exposure to jellyfish larvae, and rinse in clean seawater. Pat the body dry instead of rubbing vigorously.

In Summary

- The stinging Cnidaria of interest to Floridians are sea anemones, jellyfish, fire corals, and the Portuguese Man-of-war .
- Cnidaria have hollow, venom-filled nematocysts, which vary in length by species. Venom discharge is triggered by physical contact or by chemical stimulus.
- In Florida, jellyfish are responsible for the most marine envenomations, accounting for up to 200,000 reported stings annually.
- Increasingly common "jellyfish blooms" are thought to be triggered by climate change and poor water quality, which favor algal growth that jellyfish or their prey may feed on.
- Among the deadliest of jellyfish are the Cubozoa, which include the box jellyfish and sea wasps. Box jellyfish stings can produce Irukandji syndrome, an anaphylactic-like response.
- Sea wasps have a virulent sting that can be fatal in 15–20 percent of victims, especially young children.
- "True jellyfish" include sea nettles, lion's mane jellyfish, cannonball jellyfish, upside-down jellyfish, moon jellyfish, and thimble jellyfish. Among these, sea nettles produce the most injuries.
- The larvae of thimble jellyfish and of some of the sea anemones produce seabather's eruption, extensive and severe itching and rashes that occur when the larvae become trapped in swimwear and sting in response to the pressure of fabric against skin.
- Swimmers and divers can have encounters with two types of fire coral: branching and blade fire coral, which release nematocysts when disturbed.
- The Portuguese man-of-war is not a jellyfish but a coral-like colony of four different polyps with a tentacle reach of up to 150 feet. Stings are painful and can leave long tentacle prints of linear red streaks.
- Most Cnidaria stings are mild, producing only temporarily painful welts, swelling, and possible related itching for a few

hours or days. More severe reactions can include papules, blisters, skin necrosis, or hyperpigmentation.

- Severe allergic reactions can occur 15–30 minutes after a sting and may include low blood pressure, headache, nausea, vomiting, diarrhea, muscle spasms, fever, tightening of the chest or throat, swelling of the tongue and lips, respiratory distress, and possibly conjunctivitis, corneal ulcerations, and eyelid edema. All of these require immediate medical attention.
- Seabather's eruption is usually signaled by a tingling sensation inside of swimwear and within the cuffs of wetsuits, often while swimmers are still in the water. Rashes of dense red bumps can develop within a few hours of swimming and can be followed by severe, long-lasting itching. About a fifth of people affected report feeling generally unwell, with fevers and fatigue. Affected children may develop stomach upset.
- Treatment for almost all Cnidaria encounters usually consists of (1) neutralizing the sting with vinegar, ammonia solution, or papain; (2) removing any visible nematocysts; (3) ameliorating rashes and itching with over-the-counter topical antihistamines or corticosteroids; (4) avoiding the use of freshwater to rinse the affected area; (5) rinsing swimwear in alcohol or vinegar before washing it to help neutralize and remove nematocysts, and (6) washing and drying swimwear several times.
- Preventative measures can include wearing dive suits and gloves, wearing water shoes, applying Safe Sea sunblock, swimming with caution during summer and other jellyfish seasons, avoiding floating seaweed, removing swimwear promptly after swimming, rinsing in clean seawater, and patting dry rather than rubbing.

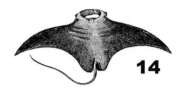

14

Doing the Stingray Shuffle

The fishermen know that the sea is dangerous and the storm
terrible, but they have never found these dangers sufficient reason
for remaining ashore.

Vincent Van Gogh

Spineless sea creatures, as we've seen, can cause problems far out
of proportion to their soft-bodied appearances. So it only stands
to reason that pokey sea creatures of greater bulk can be at least as
problematic.

In Florida, allergic reactions can occur upon contact with spine-
equipped sea creatures like stingrays, catfish, scorpionfish, and sea
urchins, among others. Between our vigorous recreational sport
fishing industry and the popularity of sunbathing, swimming, and
beachcombing in Florida, there are ample opportunities for encounters with all of these animals and their kin.

Encounters of the Fishy Kind

Although most fish allergies are dietary in nature, handling or encountering fish in their natural marine environments can also produce irritant or allergic reactions. Most reactions are due to varying
degrees of venom in fins, barbs, spines, or the slimy coat of mucus
that covers various fish species. Some reactions can occur without

the presence of venom, possibly due to the introduction of other marine irritants via puncture wounds or scratches.

Injuries and exposure can occur in any of three ways:

1. Mechanical injuries like punctures, bites, abrasions, or lacerations
2. Cutaneous (skin) exposure to dead fish or fish remains
3. Incidental skin or eye contact with allergy-triggering fish contaminants in the water[1]

By far, though, the most common trigger of allergic contact dermatitis and other reactions is encounters with spiny-rayed fish.

The Spiny-Rayed Fishes

"Spiny-rayed" fish, which may or may not be venomous but which may produce allergic and other symptoms either way, fall into five basic groups:

- Batrachoidiformes—the toadfishes
- Perciformes—the surgeonfish and stargazers in Florida
- Scorpaenidae—the lionfish, scorpionfish, and rockfish
- Siluriformes—the catfishes

While it was long believed that only about 200 species of fish were venomous, recent studies suggest the number is far higher and that perhaps as many as 2,000 ray-finned fishes may carry toxic components in their barbs and fins.[2]

Most venomous fish have grooves along their spines that facilitate defensive delivery of venom as equally into careless divers, fishermen, or beachcombers as into natural predators. Venoms have proven very similar across most species and produce a range of effects from neuromuscular to cardiovascular and everything in between. Most encounters with spiny-rayed fish result from recreational fishing, snorkeling, or scuba diving.

While catfish account for the most puncture and envenomation injuries among the spiny-rayed fish, swimmers, divers, and snorkelers around reefs and rocky areas can have painful encounters with a variety of spectacular-looking venomous fish that can send victims paddling for shore or pulling in lines in a hurry.

Toadfish (family Batrachoididae)

The toadfish, which makes its home in the Gulf of Mexico, is a remarkable and primitive-looking conglomeration of warts, stripes, and spots. Making the most of its camouflage, toadfish burrow into sandy sea bottoms to lie in wait for prey. Venomous spines along its dorsal fin and gill covers protect it from predators and deliver a nasty sting to recreational fishermen unfortunate enough to catch it, unlucky barefoot waders, or curious divers.

Toadfish venom is powerful, producing localized pain and burning, redness, and swelling. Blistering and skin necrosis may also occur.[3]

Surgeonfish and Stargazers (order Perciformes)

Surgeonfish, also known as tangs, are slender, brightly colored reef fish popular as aquarium fish. They get their name from the scalpel-like spines alongside their tail, with which they can inflict serious injury. They don't cause allergic reactions, but can cause serious injury.

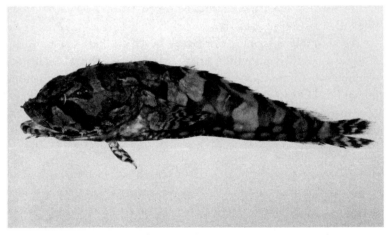

Gulf toadfish. (Photo courtesy of SEFSC Pascagoula Laboratory, collection of Brandi Noble, NOAA/NMFS/SEFSC, NOAA/USDC.)

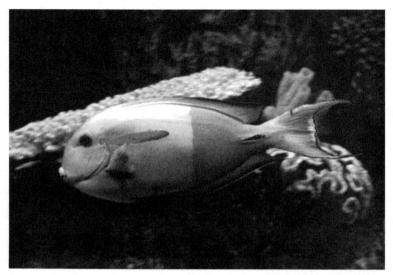

Orange-shouldered surgeonfish (*Acanthurus olivaceus*). (Photo by Lonnie Huffman, licensed under the Creative Commons Attribution 3.0 Unported license.)

When frightened, they whip their tails toward perceived danger and can lacerate a hand or a foot with, well, surgical precision. Occasionally they'll take a hook, and fishermen are cautioned to cut the line rather than try to remove the fish.[4]

The anomalous-looking stargazers, of which there are a few different species throughout the Atlantic and the Gulf of Mexico, pack a double whammy. They not only have venomous spines along their dorsal fins but can also produce an electric shock of up to 50 volts.[5] Like toadfish, they burrow in the sand to await prey. Inadvertent encounters while diving, wading, or fishing can produce painful puncture wounds that can become hot, red, and swollen.[6] The electric shock probably won't be any fun either.

Lionfish, Scorpionfish, Rockfish, and Sea Robins (order Scorpaenidae)

While scorpionfish, rockfish, and sea robins are natives, the lionfish is a new Scorpaenidae on the block. Native to the colder Indo-Pacific, the ornate-looking lionfish with its pincushion of long

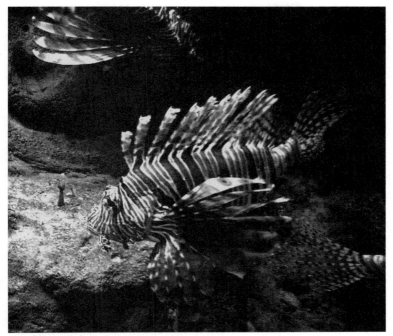

Lionfish. (Photo by Theresa Willingham.)

slender spines has been thriving in warm Florida waters throughout the Atlantic and most recently in the Gulf of Mexico since the accidental release of aquarium-kept fish, possibly dating to Hurricane Andrew in 1992.[7] While the fish are wreaking havoc on native reef fish, they're also a danger to reef divers.

Lionfish can deliver venom injections via their dorsal, anal, and pelvic fin spines, producing severe localized pain, numbness, and swelling, as well as paralysis, respiratory distress, and, rarely but on record, death.[8]

Scorpionfish, often confused with the lionfish, have shorter, frillier, fleshier spines than the lionfish and deliver a more potent venom.[9] Scorpionfish stings cause immediate throbbing pain that radiates from the point of contact, which later becomes bluish, inflamed, and hard to the touch. Physiological reactions can include sweating, paleness, respiratory problems, nausea and vomiting, diarrhea, unconsciousness, and elevated heart rates.[10]

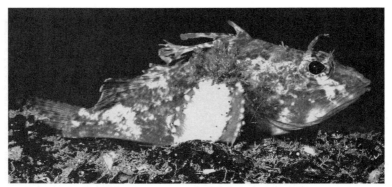

Scorpionfish. (Photo courtesy of Andrew David, NOAA/NMFS/SEFSC Panama City; Lance Horn, UNCW/NURC—Phantom II ROV operator. NOAA/ USDC.)

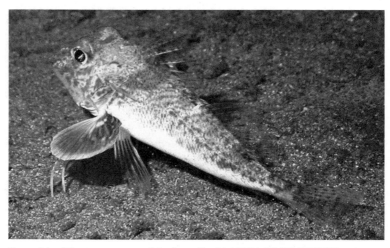

Sea robin. (Photo courtesy of Andrew David, NOAA/NMFS/SEFSC Panama City; Lance Horn, UNCW/NURC—Phantom II ROV operator. NOAA/USDC.)

Rockfish and sea robins, as alien-looking as the rest of Scorpini-dae, can also deliver a venomous sting but are generally considered less dangerous than either the scorpionfish or lionfish.

Catfish (order Siluriformes)

By far, though, the most common spiny-ray fish injuries in Florida stem from encounters with catfish. Catfish are diverse and ubiqui-

tous worldwide. There are 2,200 species of catfish across 34 taxo-
nomic families, ranging in size from the 650-pound Mekong Giant
catfish in Asia to the small walking catfish.

In Florida, catfish occur in both freshwater and saltwater environments. Principal catfish species here include the popular channel
catfish, flathead catfish, blue and white catfish, sailfin catfish, and
various bullhead catfish.[11] Popular among sport fishermen and seafood lovers alike, enjoyed by aquarium enthusiasts and treasured by
beachcombers as the "crucifix fish" for the visual suggestion in the
skeletal remains of its skull, the catfish is an integral and almost in-
escapable part of the Florida seashore environment.

But dead or alive, catfish pose a particularly pokey problem to
anyone who encounters them. Catfish get their name from the whis-
kerlike barbels common to most species. But the danger comes from
the venom-filled dorsal and pectoral spines on many catfish that lock
into an open, extended position when the fish feels threatened.[12]

Madtom, channel, and blue and white catfish are responsible
for the most injuries in the United States and, commensurately, in
Florida as well. Some catfish species also add a backup defense of

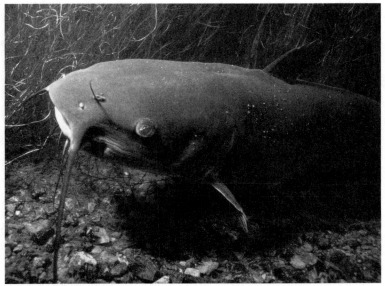

Channel catfish. (Photo by Eric Engbretson, U.S. Fish and Wildlife Service.)

protein-laden "crinotoxins" in skin secretions. Injuries can occur from handling catfish caught on a line or when waders step on live catfish (which rest with their spines erect) or step on or handle the remains of dead catfish, especially the barbs.

Most catfish-related injuries don't cause allergies, but puncture wounds can incur the need for a tetanus shot to help prevent infection from microbes in the water or on the fish.[13] Catfish venom consists of combinations of proteins that can produce constriction of blood vessels, hemolytic (blood-related) problems, or skin necrosis and which may produce intense throbbing pain that can last for up to 20 minutes. The injury site usually pales, then becomes bluish, and finally reddens and swells. Redness, neuropathy, and extensive bleeding may also occur, making for reactions that can seem far out of proportion to the size of the puncture. Victims may also experience profuse sweating and muscle spasms.[14]

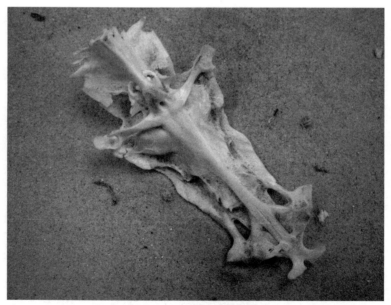

The skull of the saltwater catfish resembles the crucifixion of Christ. "The Legend of the Crucifix Fish" by Conrad S. Lantz can be found on postcards published for the Florida tourist industry.

Treating Spiny-Ray Fish Injuries

Most spiny-ray fish injuries are treated in a similar fashion:

- Clean the wound thoroughly.
- Encourage bleeding (to a safe degree) to cleanse the wound of toxins.
- Remove barb pieces as able.
- Soak the wound in hot water for 30–90 minutes.
- Get a tetanus shot if needed.[15]

It's usually recommended that the wound be left open, kept clean, and sutured at a later date if needed. Antibiotics are often prescribed as well.

Preventing Spiny-Ray Fish Injuries

Preventing injuries is often best achieved by exercising safety in and around the water. That includes wearing sturdy wading shoes, using safe handling procedures or wearing gloves when handling fish, and taking standard precautions when diving to avoid touching or annoying fish that will protect themselves in various and usually unpleasant ways. Waders should also shuffle their feet when walking through sandy areas to flush bottom dwellers like stargazers and rockfish from hiding places and help keep them out from underfoot.

The Elasmobranchs

Elasmobranchs are cartilaginous fish—meaning they have a soft inner skeleton composed of connective tissue rather than hard bone. The Elasmobranchii subclass includes sharks, skates, and rays. The spiny dogfish and stingrays are the main members of this group of interest here, because it's pretty obvious that you have more to worry about with sharks than an allergic reaction. (For the record, shark attacks in Florida waters are comparatively rare with respect to the numbers of swimmers and divers. More people drown by a factor of 20 to 1 than are bitten by sharks, and of 55 million tourists in 2001, an infinitesimal 25 or so were attacked by sharks.)[16]

The spiny dogfish is actually a type of shark, albeit one more often bitten by man than the other way around. Spiny dogfish are the only venomous shark but are nonetheless a commercially popular fish and have been in danger of being overfished. Ironically, they're also something of a nuisance fish in some areas where, true to their "dog pack" style of schooling by the thousands, they foul fishermen's nets as unwanted by-catch.[17] More important to our purposes are the spines on their dorsal fins, which can pack a venomous punch.

By far, though, more injuries occur from stingrays—up to 1,500 annually—than any other elasmobranch species.[18] Injuries are usually a result of inadvertent human blundering rather than because of any intent on the stingray's part. Notwithstanding the stingray-induced cardiac arrest death of Australian TV wild animal wrangler Steve Irwin in 2006, most stingray injuries are similar to those produced by spiny-ray fish.

There are several different types of rays living in Florida waters in both freshwater and saltwater environments. While they can vary greatly in size, color, and appearance, most rays generally resemble a stealth jet—flat, triangular, sleek, and smooth. Most have a long whiplike tail, and many are armed with a venom-filled barb at the base of the tail. Stingrays can be "benthic" (bottom dwelling) or "pelagic" (free swimming).

Benthic rays include the Atlantic stingray, the yellow and the southern stingrays. Pelagic rays are often much larger, like eagle rays and the enormous manta ray, whose "wing span" can reach over 12 feet across. Not all rays have spines. Manta rays (also known as devil rays), butterfly rays, and guitar fish are barbless elasmobranchs.[19] But along the base of the tail of many rays is a sharp, serrated spine, or barb, encased in a fleshy, often venomous sheath.

Injuries in Florida usually occur when waders step on a benthic ray buried in the sand, a common protective practice for the rays. The most common culprit is the southern stingray, which can have up to four barbs on a long tail that it lashes in self-defense.[20] On rare occasions, if the barb makes contact with a foot or leg, it can break off in the skin.[21] More often, though, it simply provokes great pain and encourages retreat. Fishermen can also be injured on the hands or arms when trying to release a hooked or netted ray. Wading inju-

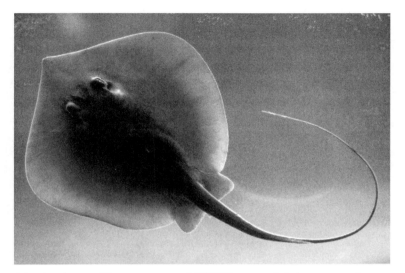

Atlantic stingray. (Photo courtesy of SEFSC Pascagoula Laboratory, collection of Brandi Noble, NOAA/NMFS/SEFSC, NOAA/USDC.)

ries usually occur between May and October, when rays are breeding and abundant.

Steve Irwin's death occurred when he swam too close to a large pelagic ray that swung its tail upward and impaled him in the heart with its barb. While not unprecedented, it was an extremely rare incident and only the third reported death by a stingray attack in Australian history. Localized tissue damage is the more common result of a stingray encounter, and occasionally there is an allergic-type reaction to the venom.

Stingray venoms contain serotonin and a couple of different types of enzymes. The serotonin induces teeth-clenching pain, and the enzymes are responsible for the tissue necrosis common in stingray injuries. Depending on the extent of injury, reactions can include a drop in blood pressure, vomiting, diarrhea, sweating, irregular heartbeat, muscle paralysis, anxiety, headache, and skin rash. Some of these symptoms may be due to an allergic reaction, others to the trauma of injury and still others can be physiological reactions to the stingray venom.[22]

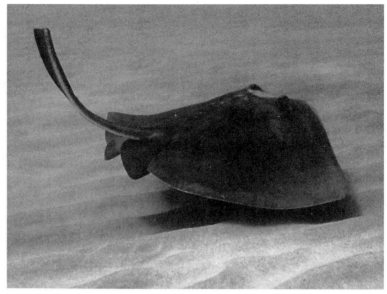

Southern stingray. (Photo by Becky A. Dayhuff, Environmental Educator, courtesy of NOAA/USDC.)

Treating Stingray Injuries

Due to the intense pain of a stingray strike, most people wisely seek medical care immediately. A tetanus shot is usually in order if one isn't current. Other basic premedical treatment can include

- removing tissue or barb fragments, unless the barb is deeply embedded and may have penetrated a blood vessel or vital organ, in which case it should be left in place for advanced medical care;
- immersing the wounded area in hot water for 30–90 minutes until significant pain relief is achieved; and
- cleansing the wound thoroughly but leaving it open for drainage.[23]

Seek professional medical care for deep wounds or lacerations and to evaluate the need for antibiotic treatments. Pain can last up to two days, and healing can take a couple of weeks.

Preventing Stingray Injuries

The Stingray Shuffle is the tried and true way to protect against stingray injuries in Florida waters. Many beaches sport signs reminding beachgoers to shuffle their feet as they wade, a practice that alerts stingrays to possible danger in time for them to move on—which the rays, as a nonaggressive species, prefer to do—rather than to react in self-defense.

There are other protective measures beachgoers can take:

- Stay out of the water when warned to do so by lifeguards or by signs or flags (purple flags indicate marine life hazards like jellyfish or rays).
- Avoid handling stingrays or trying to "ride" them.
- When swimming, diving, or snorkeling, stay well clear of the sea bottom to avoid disturbing basking rays.

The Echinoderms

The phylum Echinodermata, from *echinodermata,* which means "spiny skinned," includes another group of pokey sea creatures, the sea urchins and some starfish, as well as the smooth but occasionally noxious sea cucumber. Encounters with these creatures aren't as common or as problematic as those with catfish and stingrays, but speaking from experience, they can be just as painful.

Sea Urchins

Sea urchins are small, round, spine-covered sea creatures that spend their time moving slowly along the sea bottom, often in grass beds where they graze on algae, although some species eat corals, sponges, or other echinoderms like brittle stars. They can be entertaining to watch, maneuvering with a slow roll of their spines. Many species can be safely held in the palm, and they're popular in saltwater aquariums.

They vary in size and coloration and are a popular delicacy in some parts of the world. Beachcombers routinely encounter sea urchin remains along the beach, often without being aware of it, since

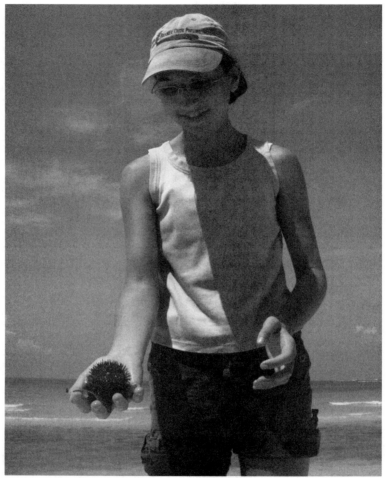

Beachgoer holding a small sea urchin. (Photo by Theresa Willingham.)

their spines drop off after they die and all that is left is a little studded oblate sphere. Many sea urchins, however, also pack a venomous punch in their spiny arsenal, the only defense they have against an array of predators for which they are also a delicacy.[24]

My sea urchin encounter was probably payback for skipping a high school class in Miami one day, and it occurred as most encounters do, while I was wading along the shore. Thrilled with our unauthorized freedom, my accomplice and I frolicked with abandon in the shallow waters along an unpopulated strip of beach off Cape Florida. The water was relatively clear, although the sandy seafloor was dotted with patches of sea grass, which I usually tried to avoid. But a high school senior recklessly skipping classes isn't likely to worry about safety, so I was thoroughly surprised by the sudden and completely unexpected shock of pain that sent me hurtling out of the water, stumbling and hopping on one foot toward shore.

My companion and I examined my foot, which was studded with several long spines, some broken, some whole, jutting out of my foot at a variety of angles. We tentatively removed those we could, but several were lodged too deeply and painfully to remove by hand. So we began the long, slow hobble back from our illusory idyll, regretting that we had hiked so far down the beach from the parking lot. I ended up in an emergency room, my pockmarked foot coated in betadine, trying to explain to my mother how I was impaled by a sea urchin when I was supposed to be in English class.

My foot throbbed for a few days, and places where spines had been embedded would flare up with hard red bumps and an intense and insistent itching for several weeks afterwards. Fortunately, I had no reactions beyond embarrassment and short-term recurrent redness and itching. And neither do most people. But as I learned, sea urchin encounters can be painful. And if spines enter joint areas, more severe problems can arise.

Venomous sea urchins injure in one of two ways, by injecting venom directly via their hollow spines or by a combination of spines and "pedicellaria," pincer-like structures at the base of each spine through which venom is released. In species with the pedicellaria, considered among the most venomous of sea urchins, the spines puncture the skin and the pedicellaria release venom into the wound.[25] Sea urchin venom contains, among other things, serotonin, proteases, and hemolytic components.[26]

Reactions can range from inflammation (especially if a spine enters near a joint), swelling and redness at the site of injury, to nausea, vomiting, numbness and tingling, muscular paralysis, nerve dysfunction, low blood pressure, or respiratory difficulties. Delayed reactions can include "tattooing" at the site of injuries caused by dark-colored sea urchins, as pigment from spines is leeched into the puncture site. Depending on the size and type of spines, they may eventually be absorbed into the skin or spontaneously extruded. Pressure on the site of injury can also cause a recurrence of pain, inflammation, burning, or itching.

Sea Cucumbers

Sea cucumbers are anomalous, squishy-looking creatures that are completely nonaggressive. They spend their days grazing along the sea bottom, gliding along with a grace belied by their generally humble looks (one local species is called the Donkey Dung sea cucumber, if that's a helpful visual).

While encounters are rare, since few people want to touch a sea cucumber anyway, they do have toxins on their bodies and in their waste that may trigger allergic contact dermatitis symptoms in some people. Mucous secretions may also cause conjunctivitis and other eye injuries and, it's been reported, blindness.[27]

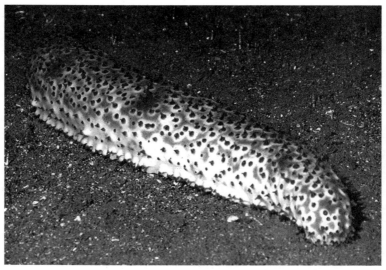

Sea cucumber. (Photo courtesy of Andrew David, NOAA/NMFS/SEFSC Panama City; Lance Horn, UNCW/NURC—Phantom II ROV operator. NOAA/USDC.)

Treating Echinoderm Injuries

On the rare chance encounter with a sea cucumber, avoid touching the creature. If it is touched, avoid touching your face afterwards. Rinse thoroughly with seawater and apply vinegar or isopropyl alcohol to the site of contact to neutralize toxins. Rinse affected eyes thoroughly with freshwater.[28]

To treat sea urchin injuries

- remove any easily graspable spines;
- immerse the wound in the hottest water you can tolerate for 30–90 minutes;
- use analgesics to alleviate pain;
- get medical care for serious reactions or for extensive injuries, including deeply embedded spines;
- see if a tetanus booster is needed, and consider prescription antibiotics to stave off infection; and
- use corticosteroids to relieve joint inflammation.[29]

Preventing Echinoderm Injuries

Echinoderms are not aggressive, nor do they injure without provocation. Injuries can usually be prevented with commonsense conduct in and around the water. Wear protective footwear when wading in shallow waters and especially through sea grasses. And don't handle or disturb sea urchins encountered while wading, diving, or snorkeling.

Mucosal Irritants

The sea cucumber isn't the only creature that can deliver passive envenomation. Some fish possess mucosal irritants. While not commonly encountered, "fish mucin hypersensitivity" presents an interesting allergenic situation for recreational or commercial fishermen and scuba divers.

A common sea bass in Florida waters, the greater soapfish, along with the white spotted and spotted soapfish (family Serranidae), secretes large amounts of a slimy mucus when disturbed, which turns into a toxic, soapy foam (hence its name). People rarely get near enough to a soapfish to provoke this kind of reaction. They are nocturnal and tend to hang out on reefs or sandy sea bottoms, leaning motionlessly against rocks. For the hapless fisherman who may pull it up on a line or the curious diver, though, soapfish secretions may prove irritating to the skin.[30]

The common bluegill (*Lepomis macrochirus*) has been found to produce a similarly irritating compound in the mucosal covering of its skin.[31] Glycoproteins seem to be the principal IgE antibody triggering allergic rhinitis, contact urticaria, and angioedema in people who handle the fish. There may be a connection between dietary fish allergy and fish contact allergy.

Like most contact allergies, sensitivity to the mucosal film on fish is best treated by prevention. If sensitivity to handling fish appears to be a problem, wearing gloves and protective clothing is the best protection.

Miscellaneous Marine Envenomators

A handful of other creatures pose potential envenomation issues for swimmers and divers in Florida waters, including the fire sponge, bristle worms, and fire worms. Their names should offer sufficient warning as to the problems they present.

Sponges (phylum Porifera)

Sponges, appearances to the contrary, are animals, not plants. The fire sponge, a particularly virulent variety, tips off divers readily about its toxicity with its bright red or orange coloration. Contact with the sponge produces an immediate burning sensation and a commensurate rash.[32] It's definitely not one for the bathtub! Papules and vesicles may also occur.[33]

Other live sponges may produce irritant skin dermatitis as well, due to the sharp silicon or calciferous spicules that make up the sponge's internal structure. Fishermen, divers, or swimmers are the most likely individuals to make contact with live sponges. Fresh specimens washed up on the beach may also produce contact dermatitis when handled. Other reactions to handling live sponges can include pain, redness, itching, and skin tingling and numbness.[34]

In a similar fashion, bryozoans, another plantlike animal occurring in freshwater or saltwater and often incidentally encountered by fishermen, can also provoke serious irritant contact dermatitis.

Avoiding injury is usually a matter of taking common sense preventative measures: not handling or touching sponges, and wearing protective gloves and clothing when diving or fishing.

Marine Annelids

Annelids, or segmented worms, which include terrestrial varieties of earthworms and leeches, also occur throughout the world's oceans and in reasonable abundance around Florida. Evoking images of miniaturized versions of the worms of Frank Herbert's novel *Dune* or the film *Tremors*, marine annelids come in many shapes and as-

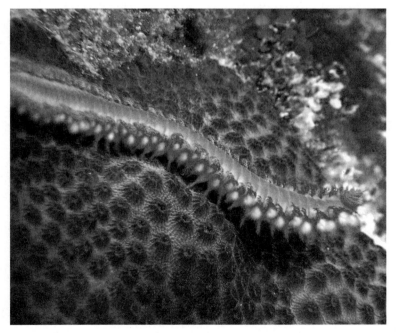

Bearded or orange fire worm, U.S. Virgin Islands. (Photo by Becky A. Dayhuff, Environmental Educator, courtesy of NOAA/USDC.)

sume a variety of defensive measures, principal among these their biting jaws and toxic stinging bristles.

Swimmers, snorkelers, and divers are the most likely to encounter the more common varieties of annelids that can injure or provoke contact irritation, mainly the blood worm and the bristle worm.

Blood worms are common throughout the Atlantic and Gulf of Mexico. Popular as bait, this bait bites back with chitinous jaws that produce a reaction reminiscent of a bee sting. The biting reef worm is a close blood worm relative that, as its name implies, will bite. As it can reach four feet in length, one may safely assume its bite is significantly more powerful and painful than that of other worms.[35]

Blood worm bites leave an oval-shaped mark with a red spot in the center. Swelling may continue for a day or two after the bite. Soaking the bite in vinegar helps alleviate pain and discomfort.

Bristle worms, of which there are several species in the Atlantic and Gulf of Mexico, include the green fire worm and the red-tipped fire worm. They can grow to 5–10 inches in length and protect themselves with detachable rows of bristles that can become lodged in the skin like cactus spines.

The spines cause itching and numbness where they contact the skin, as well as inflammation and redness. Treatment consists of removing the bristles, usually with repeated passes of adhesive tape, in the same manner that plant hair irritants are removed from the skin. A 3:1 solution of water and ammonia, or soaking in isopropyl alcohol, helps relieve pain and neutralize toxins.

Prevention is mostly a matter of not handling blood worms or bristle worms. Red-tipped fire worms may sometimes take a fisherman's hook, in which case gloves should be worn to remove the worm. Marine annelids encountered while swimming, diving, or snorkeling should be respected and left alone.

In Summary

- Contact with spiny sea creatures (spiny-rayed fish, stingrays, sea urchins, sea sponges, and annelids) or with fish sheathed in toxic mucus can produce allergic reactions.

- Injuries from marine life can be (1) mechanical (punctures, cuts, and abrasions); (2) cutaneous (through skin]exposure to dead fish or their remains); and (3) incidental (through skin or eye contact with allergy-triggering waterborne fish contaminants).
- Though similar across most species, spiny-rayed fish venoms can produce a range of effects from neuromuscular to cardio-vascular and everything in between.
- The most common spiny-ray fish injuries in Florida are caused by catfish. The protein-laden venom in their spines can produce intense throbbing pain, redness, swelling, muscle spasms, and neuropathy.
- Most spiny-ray fish injuries are treated by cleaning the wound thoroughly, encouraging bleeding to flush toxins, remov-ing any barb pieces from the skin, soaking the wound in hot water, and keeping the wound open and clean. A tetanus shot may be required.
- Spiny-ray fish injuries can be prevented by taking safety precautions in and around the water, including wearing sturdy wading shoes, wearing gloves when handling fish, and refrain-ing from touching or annoying fish while diving.
- Up to 1,500 stingray injuries occur annually, usually between May and October when rays are breeding. Stingrays are "ben-thic" (bottom dwelling) or "pelagic" (swimming), and most injuries in Florida occur when waders step on a benthic ray, usually the southern stingray, buried in the sand.
- Stingray injury reactions, either allergic or trauma-induced, can include a drop in blood pressure, vomiting, diarrhea, sweating, irregular heartbeat, muscle paralysis, anxiety, head-ache, and skin rash.
- Basic treatment of stingray injuries involves removing easily accessible tissue or barb fragments, immersing the wounded area in hot water for 30–90 minutes until significant pain re-lief is achieved, cleansing the wound thoroughly, and leaving it open for drainage.
- The Stingray Shuffle—shuffling the feet while wading—is the

best way to ward off stingrays and prevent injuries. Other protective measures include observing marine life hazard warnings, not handling stingrays, and staying well clear of the sea bottom when swimming, diving, or snorkeling.

- Sea urchins cause injury by injecting venom into the skin through their hollow spines and, sometimes, through the pincer-like "pedicellaria" at the base of the spines.

- Reactions to sea urchin injuries can include inflammation, especially if a spine enters near a joint, swelling and redness at the injury site, nausea, vomiting, numbness and tingling, muscular paralysis, nerve dysfunction, low blood pressure, and respiratory difficulties. Delayed reactions can include "tattooing" (where pigment from a dark sea urchin enters the skin at the puncture site) as well as synovitis and granuloma, where pieces of spine are trapped under the skin.

- Treat sea urchin injuries by removing any easily graspable spines, immersing the wound in the hottest water tolerable for 30–90 minutes, taking analgesics as needed, and seeking medical care for extensive injuries.

- Sea urchin injuries can be prevented by wearing protective footwear when wading in shallow waters, avoiding sea grasses, and not handling or disturbing sea urchins.

- "Fish mucin hypersensitivity" is an allergic response to the mucosal film of some fish species (soapfish and bluegill, for example) and is most commonly experienced by recreational or commercial fishermen and some divers. Sensitivity to the mucosal fluids is best avoided by wearing gloves and protective clothing when handling fish.

- Other sea creatures that can cause allergic reactions include sponges and marine worms, whose spicules, bristles, and bites can irritate the skin. Prevention of injury can be achieved by wearing protective gloves and appropriate dive gear and by not handling the animals.

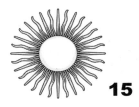

15

Sun and Sea
A Day at the Beach

Praise the sea; on shore remain.

John Florio

Florida is all about water. Visitors and residents alike enjoy nearly 6,000 liquid square miles along more than 2,000 miles of tidal shoreline (8,400 "detailed" miles), 12,000 miles of rivers, streams, and waterways, and 3 million acres of lakes in which to swim, dive, snorkel, fish, boat, and play.[1] Most of the time, Florida waters are paradise on Earth.

Sugar sand beaches invite sunbathing and beachcombing. Warm Atlantic and Gulf of Mexico waters are made to order for swimming, windsurfing, jet skiing, sailing, and fishing. A family entertainment mecca, Florida's hotels feature pools and hot tubs, and there are dozens of water theme parks throughout the state, with waterslides, man-made lagoons, and kiddie pools.

Unless, of course, you get sunburn or suffer from photoallergic dermatitis or "sun allergy." And then sometimes our liquid Eden can become hell on Earth, a splash through the veritable River Styx.

For all our water and all our sunshine provide a rich growing medium for a variety of algae, bacteria, and other organisms that can produce allergenic and other irritating symptoms when they "bloom." Seventy of the estimated 100 toxic algae species that cause harmful algal blooms, or HABs, occur in Florida waters.[2]

Some of the algae are potentially toxic to fish or shellfish, but haven't been shown to cause any ill effects to people. Others, like the dinoflagellates that produce red tide, can not only cause fish kills but produce water and airborne toxins that cause respiratory problems in humans.

Besides algae, there are sundry and diverse bacterial, fungal and other conditions that can produce Recreational Water Illnesses, or RWIs, which can include things like *Cryptosporidium*-induced GI problems and "swimmer's itch."

Let's start on the beach and then go test the waters.

Photosensitivity

Most people will never encounter anything more serious from a day at the beach than sunburn, a problem that can be prevented by dressing appropriately and using adequate sunscreen protection of Sun Protection Factor (SPF) 15 (which filters out 92 percent of harmful ultraviolet B wavelength radiation) or higher. For some people, though, especially those with fair skin and light-colored hair, people taking certain medications, or those with conditions like systemic lupus erythematosus, exposure to the ultraviolet radiation of sunlight can produce photosensitivity.[3]

Also known as photoallergic dermatitis, sun poisoning, or sun allergy, this is a delayed hypersensitivity to sunlight that usually results from either a combination of an allergen and sunlight or an autoimmune disorder. Other risk factors can include ethnicity—light-skinned individuals are more prone to sun-related skin problems like atopic dermatitis—existing skin conditions, and genetic history.[4]

Five basic types of photosensitivity can occur:

- Solar urticaria produces hives within a few minutes of exposure to sunlight. The hives usually last only a few hours but can be accompanied by headaches, dizziness, and sensations of weakness and nausea.
- Actinic prurigo, more common in children and young adults

and among Native Americans, can produce red, raised patches of skin and itchy bumps that may become blisters that crack open. The eruption can extend to areas of skin that weren't exposed to sunlight and can cause chapped split lips and affect areas of the face, neck, arms, and hands. This may leave scarring.

- Chronic actinic dermatitis is more extensive in nature, with symptoms similar to that of allergic contact dermatitis. It can cause thick patches of dry, itchy, and inflamed skin, sometimes with "islands" of unaffected skin, on the face, arms, hands, and upper torso.

- Chemical photosensitivity is the result of sunlight exposure in combination with the use of certain medications, like tetracycline, or certain perfumes or other skin applications that make the skin more sensitive to UV light. Those subject to chemical photosensitivity can experience itchy hives, redness, inflammation, and sometimes brown or blue skin discoloration.

- Polymorphous light eruption (PMLE) is among the most common but least understood sun-related skin eruptions. It's more common in women and presents as multiple red bumps and irregular red areas of open skin within 30 minutes to several hours after sun exposure. New patches of reddened areas can occur hours to days later. Reactions usually disappear within several days to a week after initial exposure and tend to diminish with gradually increasing exposure to the sun.[5]

Diagnosing Photosensitivity

While it may not seem like rocket science to diagnose a sunlight-induced condition, so many things can cause skin reactions that it's important to winnow out other factors. The most common ways to diagnose photosensitivity are UV light testing, or phototesting, which evaluates skin responses to different wavelengths of light; photopatch testing, which tests to see if there are certain chemicals or medications that might be making the skin react to sunlight; and, rarely, blood tests and skin samples.

Photosensitivity Treatments and Prevention

Treatments include standard sunburn salves, applying a cold compress, cooling gels, or ointments, and taking aspirin or acetaminophen to relieve discomfort or inflammation. Those suffering from polymorphous light eruption or lupus photosensitivity are sometimes treated with oral or topical corticosteroids. Phototherapy, which can help desensitize the skin to ultraviolet light, can also be helpful.

There are several preventative measures those sensitive to sunlight can (and everyone should anyway!) employ for maximum safety in the Florida sun:

- Take appropriate precautions like using sunscreen and wearing protective clothing and sunglasses when outdoors during periods of peak UV exposure, usually between 10 am and 4 pm.
- People highly sensitive to sunlight should wear lightweight, light-colored long-sleeved shirts and a hat that shades the neck area.
- Avoid tanning beds and sunbathing.
- Apply SPF 15 or higher sunscreen, even on cloudy days, 20 minutes before going outdoors and every two hours while outside, as well as immediately after swimming or vigorous activity.

Now that you've got your hat and sunscreen on, let's take a look at the water.

Harmful Algal Blooms

Algae are simple, plantlike organisms that are autotrophic—able to synthesize their own food from sunlight or inorganic substances. Although they can utilize photosynthesis, they differ from plants in cellular makeup, and by their lack of leaves, roots, and other common plant organs. Algae range from small, single-celled dinoflagellates to intricate multicellular, fast-growing seaweed forms like the Pacific giant kelp that grows in dense marine "forests" and can reach lengths of more than 100 feet.[6]

Algae are mostly harmless and deeply vital "primary" producers upon which much of the world's food chain is built. They create oxygen and provide the basis of many medicines, foods, and products ranging from cosmetics to cleaners. And just as cancer cells are ordinarily useful cells run amok, harmful algal blooms (HABs)—the scientifically more accurate and preferred term for water conditions like "red tide"—occur when certain species of algae reproduce in counterproductive overabundance. Blooms can deplete oxygen, cut off sunlight required by other organisms, and release toxins into the air and water. Some scientists believe blooms are increasing because of climate change conditions, although most evidence suggests that nutrient-rich runoff is the biggest culprit.[7]

In Florida, three basic types of algae can cause health problems in people:

- Cyanobacteria, a blue-green algae responsible for freshwater HABs
- Dinoflagellates, motile algae that can cause fish kills and produce both water and airborne toxins to which people can be sensitive
- Diatoms, a silicon-based phytoplankton

Cyanobacteria—Allergy/Irritant potential: High

Cyanobacteria, also known as blue-green algae, are among the oldest living things on earth. Consequently, they're pretty primitive in design, lacking the internal structures of related diatoms and dinoflagellates. The twenty or so species of blue-green algae in Florida can produce three major types of toxins: hepatotoxins, affecting the liver; neurotoxins, affecting the nervous system; and dermatoxins, irritating the skin.

Whether because of its primordial nature or because of kelp's strong resemblance to overgrown spinach, blue-green algae in the form of spirulina or *Aphanizomenon flos-aquae* (AFA) is also touted by some as good for everything from weight loss to curing cancer. Studies, however, suggest otherwise. In fact, blue-green algae supplements have been found to have high levels of a hepatoxin called microcystin.[8]

Misguided health enthusiasts needn't look far for blue-green algae in Florida. Cyanobacteria is common in our fresh and brackish water habitats where, under certain circumstances, it can undergo blooms, or "scums," killing fish and creating an overabundance of natural toxins.[9]

Depending on the extent of a bloom, either a thick, sometimes smelly pond scum can develop, or the bloom can disperse in the water, turning it a vivid shade of green, brown, and sometimes red. Nutrient-rich runoff from overfertilized fields and lawns is a suspected culprit in the blooms. People exposed to the blooms can suffer gastrointestinal distress, itchy rashes, and other symptoms from inhaling, touching, or ingesting organic components of the blooms.[10]

Anabaena circinalis and *Microcystis aeruginosa* are the most common types of cyanobacteria in Florida and are responsible for most of the blooms in lakes and ponds during the warm season. *Microcystis* is particularly pervasive, making its way into drinking water reservoirs nationwide. It's been found in 80 percent of more than 600 water samples taken from 45 utility companies around the country, 4 percent of which exceeded World Health Organization safety recommendations.

One species of cyanobacteria, called *Lyngbya majuscule,* produces severe dermatitis on contact and GI problems if ingested. It is suspected in complaints of rashes and skin irritation reported in Florida parks with spring-fed streams, although the Florida Department of Health Aquatoxins Department has found no evidence of the cyanobacteria in water samples. While most dermatologic reports remain anecdotal, Type I hypersensitivity to cyanobacteria has been reported with exposure to recreational water contaminated with the algae.[11]

Cyanotoxicity

Cyanotoxicity, illness, or allergenic-type reactions stemming from exposure to cyanobacteria can result from accidental ingestion of contaminated water while swimming, drinking contaminated water, inhaling airborne cyanotoxins, and touching cyanobacteria. Symptoms of cyanotoxicity, which can occur up to 36 hours after exposure, can be extensive. According to G. Meghan Abbott and her colleagues at the Florida Fish and Wildlife Conservation Commission, reactions include

- rash, hives, or blisters, particularly around the face and under swimsuits;
- allergic rhinitis;
- respiratory problems, including asthma-like symptoms;
- sore throat;
- acute gastroenteritis;
- liver or kidney toxicity; and
- neurologic effects, like salivation and muscle cramps, twitching, paralysis, and cardiac or respiratory failure.[12]

Diagnosis of cyanotoxicity is based on a clinical evaluation and a history of exposure. Samples of the water to which one has been exposed can facilitate diagnosis. And studies are under way to find ways to detect cyanotoxins in the blood.

Treatment of Cyanotoxicity

Treatment typically consists of eliminating exposure and providing supportive treatment for symptoms. Activated carbon can be administered for incidents of ingestion. People at higher risk of developing cyanotoxicity include young children, the elderly, and those with existing immunologic, neurologic, liver, or kidney disease.

Prevention is the most effective way of avoiding cyanotoxins, and precautions can be taken even if HAB warnings are not in effect or are missed. Preventative measures include

- avoiding contact with water if algae are visible in the form of foam, scum, or mats;
- avoiding or limiting swimming, boating, or other recreational activities near or on water during periods of algal blooms; and
- rinsing with freshwater immediately after exposure.[13]

Pets can be at high risk of exposure and fatal reactions, and they should be kept out of contaminated waters and washed immediately if exposed to cyanobacteria. While cyanotoxicity is not a reportable disease in Florida, the Florida Department of Health asks health-care providers to report suspected cases to the Aquatic Toxin Hotline at 1-888-232-8635 or the Aquatic Toxins Program at www.myfloridaeh.com.

Flagellates—Allergy/Irritant Potential: High

Flagellates are a single-celled step up from cyanobacteria, with organic cell walls and the capability of locomotion via their whiplike flagella, from which their name is derived. Up to 70 percent of HABs are caused by dinoflagellates, so called for the "whirling" (Greek *dinos*) motion of their flagella, which gives them mostly vertical mobility.

Parting the Red Tide: *Karenia brevis*

Red tide, the most recognizable of the flagellate-induced HABs, is caused by the dinoflagellate *Karenia brevis*, or *K. brevis*. Red tide is not new in Florida. Reports of the phenomenon in the Gulf of Mexico date back to the 1500s. It traditionally occurs in the late summer and early fall, usually in the Gulf Coast between Clearwater and Sanibel Island. Although far less common, red tide has also been known to occur in the Atlantic Ocean.

Red tide is particularly striking for the breadth and duration of the bloom, which, at its worst, can occur sporadically for more than a year and affect thousands of square miles, killing countless fish, birds and marine mammals in its path.[14] In March 2011, the National Institute of Environmental and Health Sciences released the results of the largest red tide study ever conducted. As expected, the study found that *Karenia brevis* contains at least a dozen harmful toxins, known as brevetoxins. But the study also uncovered three useful antitoxins in the algae.[15]

One of these newly discovered antitoxins is being used in the development of a new cystic fibrosis drug called Brevenal and has possible applications in treating chronic obstructive pulmonary disease and other ailments. But most people will only experience the less positive effects of this HAB.

In many parts of Florida, red tide is a seasonal part of coastal life. On a visit to Siesta Key one fall, our seaside stroll turned somber when we came upon signs warning of red tide. Dead fish of every variety littered the waterline, where they were set upon by hundreds of seabirds.

The odor wasn't immediately apparent because of offshore breezes, but when the wind changed, the smell and the brevetoxins provoking coughs and watery eyes were sufficient to drive us off the beach. Surprisingly, despite signs and stench, diehard beachgoers were undeterred and happily engaged in windsurfing, parasailing, and swimming even as fish continued to wash ashore.

Bravado in the face of brevetoxins isn't such a good idea. Brevetoxins can affect people in several ways, including neurotoxic shellfish poisoning (NSP) or paralytic shellfish poisoning from eating affected shellfish, respiratory distress (red tide cough) from inhaled toxins, and contact dermatitis.

Neurotoxic Shellfish Poisoning (NSP)

While not an allergy, this unfortunate by-product of red tide bears mentioning. NSP is not usually encountered in restaurants, since commercial establishments typically ensure safety in their shellfish. But diners eating locally harvested shellfish can accidentally expose themselves to NSP. Because they're filter-feeders, clams, oysters, and mussels can accumulate brevetoxins during a red tide bloom that then affect those who eat them.

Symptoms, which can begin up to 18 hours after ingestion, are what would be expected in cases of food poisoning. They can include vomiting, diarrhea, stomach pain, numbness and tingling in the lips, mouth, face, and extremities, loss of feeling and control of the legs, and difficulty breathing.[16]

Diagnosis of NSP is usually based on clinical presentation and a patient history of recent consumption of shellfish. Numbness and tingling around the face and in the extremities are the most commonly reported symptoms. Treatment consists primarily of supportive care, although activated charcoal can be helpful within the first four hours. Most people recover within a couple of days, and there have been no reported fatalities or long-term effects from NSP.

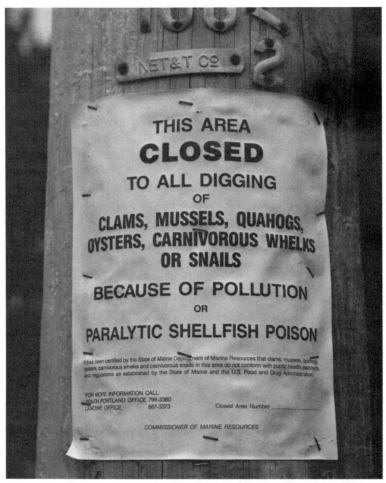

Paralytic shellfish poisoning warning signs like this one appear in areas that have been closed due to high levels of toxin in shellfish and should be heeded. (Photo courtesy of National Ocean Service, NOAA/USDC.)

Red Tide Cough

Brevetoxins can become aerosolized—suspended in the air—through sea spray from waves or splashing, and when inhaled they can produce brevetoxin-associated respiratory syndrome, more commonly called "red tide cough."[17] Those with sinusitis, asthma, or other respiratory disorders are most susceptible, but anyone can potentially be sensitive to aerosolized brevetoxins.

Symptoms can occur within minutes of exposure and linger for days, producing a dry cough, sneezing, watery eyes, shortness of breath or wheezing, and a sensation of chest constriction. Symptoms are usually exacerbated in direct proportion to beach proximity, especially on red tide days with an onshore breeze. There have also been reports of tinnitus, itchiness, and dizziness.

As with NSP, diagnosis is usually based on a clinical evaluation and medical history of symptoms and exposure. Treatment typically consists of retreating indoors, into a climate-controlled location, and remaining away from affected areas, especially during periods of onshore winds.

Studies are under way to evaluate the effects of bronchodilators to ameliorate or reverse the effects of inhaled brevetoxins. In the meantime, dust or particle masks can be helpful if going outdoors during a red tide event is unavoidable.

Red Tide Contact Dermatitis

Although it's rarely reported—perhaps because the sore throat, coughing, and sneezing and the aroma of dead fish on the beach are enough to keep most people out of the water—red tide–induced contact dermatitis can occur. Typically, it appears as a rash after swimming in or contacting contaminated water, but it goes away within 24 hours. Rinsing immediately after exposure to red tide waters reduces the chances of developing dermatitis.

Pfiesteria piscicida

Pfiesteria piscicida and the related *Pseudopfiesteria shumwayae* are dinoflagellates that have been responsible for producing ulcerations on fish on both coasts. While there are no reports of widespread blooms or fish kills from either species here in Florida, and they aren't thought to be a public health threat at this time, the Florida Fish and Wildlife Conservation Commission considers *pfiesteria* a species of concern due to problems caused by the flagellates in other eastern seaboard states.[18]

As a result, the state monitors waters for blooms and reports of related ill health, called pfiesteriosis, which can be triggered by skin contact or inhalation of *pfiesteria* toxin. Symptoms of pfiesteriosis, which can be produced from small doses of the toxin, can include

- eye irritation and long-term vision problems;
- respiratory problems;
- nausea;
- disorientation, confusion, irritability, or mood swings;
- headaches;
- skin lesions and rashes;
- kidney and liver problems; and
- immune system problems.[19]

While there have been no reports of illness from eating contaminated shellfish or seafood, researchers recommend avoiding contact or consumption of fish showing lesions or caught in *pfiesteria* contaminated waters.

Diatoms—Allergy/Irritant Potential: Mild

Diatoms are phytoplankton, and they differ from blue-green algae and dinoflagellates by virtue of their silicate-based composition. Because they require silica to grow, diatoms don't bloom as often or as abundantly as the more opportunistic cyanobacteria or dinoflagellates.[20] However, because of their very specific nutrient needs, they're a good indicator of water health and can provide evidence of silicate contamination wherever blooms occur.

Diatom blooms have occurred periodically over the last 20 years near freshwater outflows in the Florida Bay, along the Gulf of Mexico, and most recently in the spring of 2009 along the Flagler, Volusia, and Brevard county coastlines, where bathers reported "slick" and foamy brown water with a bad odor.[21] There were also reports of red tide–like throat irritation and respiratory problems.

Researchers identified diatoms hailing from the genus *Thalassiosira*, which naturally form large gelatinous colonies that drift in the open ocean and can sometimes be brought ashore by the Gulf Stream. The diatom blooms can kill fish by clogging their gills and lowering oxygen in the water where a bloom occurs. The Fish and

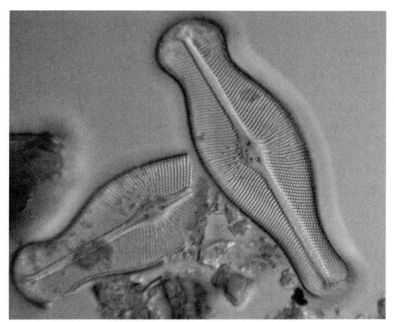

Diatom *Didymosphenia geminata* cell wall description: Image of the silica cell wall of the diatom *Didymosphenia geminata* from Rio Espolon, Chile. The sample was collected early in 2010 from an extensive bloom on the river. The image has been processed to show the silica cell wall, removing the organic cell contents and the stalk material. (Photo by Sarah Spaulding, USGS.)

Wildlife Commission continues to monitor diatom blooms on both coasts of Florida.

Recreational Water Illness (RWI)

Recreational Water Illnesses, or RWIs, are a bit more amorphous than algae blooms. They're spread by contact, ingestion, or inhalation of waters in public or residential pools, fountains, hot tubs, ponds, or lakes contaminated by various types of bacteria or algae. While the most commonly reported RWI is diarrhea, other symptoms can include eye and wound infections, respiratory problems, and dermatitis.[22]

For obvious reasons, Florida ranks among the top states for RWIs in the nation. Other top contenders are California and various northeastern states. (In 2005 in New York, 1,800 people became sick after visiting a water park in Seneca.)[23] While most RWIs are not technically "allergies," many can cause contact dermatitis and allergy-like respiratory problems, and visitors and residents alike should be familiar with them. RWIs are best understood by looking at the contamination environment.

Pools and Water Parks—Most Common Contaminant: Parasites

There are well over a million residential pools in Florida, hundreds of municipal pools, dozens of public water parks, and in recent years "spraygrounds" decked out with water fountains and squirters instead of swings and slides. Recreational water in pools and fountains, especially that in which young children play, can be easily contaminated with fecal material bearing the parasites *Cryptosporidium* or *Giardia intestinalis*, as well as other pathogens like *Norovirus* and *E. coli*, if chlorine levels aren't properly maintained.

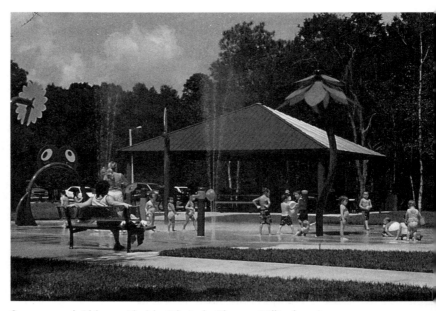

Sprayground, Oldsmar, Florida. (Photo by Theresa Willingham.)

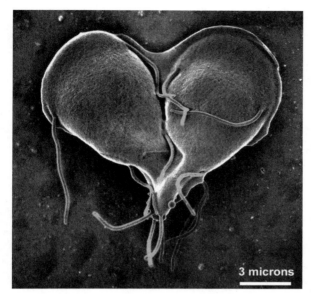

This scanning electron micrograph (SEM) shows a *Giardia lamblia* protozoan caught in a late stage of cell division, producing a heart-shaped form. The protozoan *Giardia* causes the diarrheal disease called giardiasis. (Photo by Dr. Stan Erlandsen, CDC.)

Ingesting water contaminated by either or both parasites can cause diarrhea and other GI problems. In 2005–2006, the CDC collated nearly 60 reported cases of cryptosporidiosis and *Giardia*-related illness in Florida pools. Countless numbers go unreported because people may not make the connection about how they become ill.

The Florida Department of Health recommends some basic safety precautions for avoiding crypto and giardiasis:

- Keep sick children (and adults) away from public bathing areas.
- Avoid swallowing water from pools and interactive fountains.
- Shower with soap and water, and wash children well before and after swimming.
- Do not change diapers poolside, and wash hands well after changing or handling diapers.
- Give children frequent restroom breaks and check diapers often.

Hot Tubs—Most Common Contaminant:
Bacterium *Pseudomonas aeruginosa*

Most people slip into a hot tub or spa seeking relaxation. But if the water isn't properly maintained, it's not too hard to come out with a rash instead. "Hot tub rash" is a type of dermatitis triggered by the bacteria *Pseudomonas aeruginosa*.[24] The bacteria proliferate in poorly maintained spas and hot tubs and can produce tender, itchy red bumps and pus-filled blisters near hair follicles, known as *Pseudomona* folliculitis. Appearances to the contrary, *Pseudomona* folliculitis is not an allergic reaction but a bacterial colonization of the hair follicles.[25]

Rashes may be worse in areas covered by a swimsuit, possibly because of trapped contaminated water in those areas. Vigorous rubbing while in the water facilitates bacterial infection, which may explain the preponderance of water slide induced cases. Problems are also exacerbated by low pH, hot water, and commensurate low chlorine levels, possibly because chlorine dissipates more quickly in hot temperatures. Respiratory problems have also been reported as a result of poorly maintained hot tubs.

Mild cases usually clear up of their own accord, but recurring or persistent problems should be evaluated by a medical professional. To reduce chances of developing hot tub rash, limit time spent in hot tubs, maintain safe pH and chlorine levels, and keep hot tub temperatures below 105 degrees.[26]

Lakes, Rivers, and Ponds—Most Common Contaminants:
Parasites and Amoebas

As with pools, disease-causing organisms can contaminate lakes, ponds, and rivers from sewage, animal waste, and runoff. Heavy rainfalls increase the chances of bacterial infection from local water bodies, as does swimming during hot summer months.

Cryptosporidium and *Giardia intestinalis*, the aforementioned parasites that cause diarrhea, are among the most commonly encountered sources of illness in Florida lakes and ponds. But a more disturbing condition has come to the forefront: primary amoebic meningoencephalitis caused by the amoeba *Naegleri fowleri*, or *N. fowleri*.

A rare but increasingly reported illness with a 95 percent mortality rate, amoebic disease occurs when swimmers jump or dive into warm freshwater or stagnant ponds or lakes. Jumping into waters where *N. fowleri* lives forces the amoeba up into the nose, from which it travels into the brain causing death within a week as a result of swelling and fluid build-up in the brain.[27]

N. fowleri normally lives unnoticed in nearly half of Florida's lakes. Springs are considered safe because water temperatures remain below 80 degrees. About 25 cases of primary amoebic meningoencephalitis have been documented in Florida, three in recent years in recreational waters in Central Florida, where teens have died after playing in ski parks and local ponds.

Swimmers can reduce their chances of acquiring primary amoebic meningoencephalitis in several ways:

- Stay out of warm freshwater, hot springs, or thermally polluted water, such as that found near power plants.
- Avoid stagnant water.
- Use nose clips when swimming in freshwater ponds and lakes.
- Avoid digging in or stirring up sediment in shallow, warm freshwater environments.

Swimmer's Itch—Contaminant: Parasites

Similar to seabather's eruption, swimmer's itch, also known as cercarial dermatitis, is a skin rash caused by an allergic reaction to microscopic parasites occurring in freshwater and saltwater. The parasites, which are dispersed by infected snails, typically prefer bird or mammal hosts but will infect humans, burrowing into the skin and triggering rashes and itching.[28]

Symptoms of swimmer's itch can occur within minutes to hours of swimming in contaminated water and may include skin tingling, burning, or itching and small reddish pimples or blisters.

Itching can last a week or more, and excessive scratching can produce secondary infections. Because cercarial dermatitis is an allergic reaction, the more often a sensitive individual swims in infected waters, the more severe and immediate commensurate reactions tend to be.

Treatment is usually aimed at relieving symptoms and can include applications of corticosteroid creams, calamine lotion or cool compresses; soaking in baking soda, colloidal oatmeal, or Epson salt solutions; and taking antihistamines.

Swimmer's itch can be avoided in several ways:

- Avoid contact with water in marshy areas where snails are common.
- Avoid waters known to harbor potentially problematic snails.
- Discourage birds in public bathing areas.
- Shower or rinse off immediately after swimming.

Most RWIs are considered "nonreportable" illnesses, meaning doctors and hospitals aren't required to report potential cases of water-borne illnesses as such. However, the Florida Fish and Wildlife Research Institute welcomes citizen reports and recommends contacting them at 1-800-232-8635 to report symptoms from Florida red tide or any suspected aquatic toxin.

In Summary

- Fair-skinned people with light hair may develop photosensitivity, also called photoallergic dermatitis, sun poisoning, and sun allergy; it is a delayed hypersensitivity usually to a combination of an allergen and sunlight or from an autoimmune disorder.
- Five basic types of photosensitivity are: (1) solar urticaria, with short-term hives; (2) actinic prurigo, more common in children, young adults, and Native Americans, causing red, raised patches and itchy bumps, extensive chapping, and possible scarring; (3) chronic actinic dermatitis, with symptoms similar to allergic contact dermatitis; (4) chemical photosensitivity, a reaction to sunlight exposure and use of certain medications; and (5) polymorphous light eruption (PMLE), the most common but least understood of sun-related skin eruptions, occurring most often in women.
- Treatments for photosensitivity include standard sunburn

treatments, oral or topical corticosteroids, and sometimes phototherapy.

- Precautions against photosensitivity involve dressing appropriately, applying SPF 15 or higher sunscreen, avoiding peak hours of UV exposure, and not sunbathing or using tanning beds.
- The two basic categories of waterborne irritants in Florida are harmful algae blooms (HABs) and recreational water illnesses (RWIs).
- HABs are usually caused by three basic algae: cyanobacteria, dinoflagellates, and diatoms.
- Cyanobacteria, or blue-green algae, occur in freshwater and brackish environments as the result of nutrient-rich run-off. They produce cyanotoxins that can affect the liver, nervous system, and skin.
- The dinoflagellate *K. brevis* causes red tide, which produces brevetoxins responsible for neurotoxic shellfish poisoning (NSP) and red tide cough.
- NSP from eating contaminated shellfish can cause tingling of the face and extremities, vomiting, diarrhea, and stomach pain. Red tide cough involves a dry cough, sneezing, watery eyes, and shortness of breath.
- Diatom blooms, the least common and shortest-lived of the HABs, turn water slick, foamy, and brown with a strong odor that triggers red tide–like respiratory problems and throat irritation.
- HAB exposure symptoms can be ameliorated by staying indoors during periods of algae or diatom blooms, avoiding beach areas when an offshore breeze is blowing, or wearing a face mask.
- RWIs are often parasitic or bacterial diseases spread through contact with fecal-contaminated public recreational pools, water parks and fountains. The most commonly reported RWIs are *Cryptosporidium*- and *Giardia*-induced diarrhea.
- Crypto and giardiasis are best avoided by keeping sick children from public bathing areas; not swallowing water in

public bathing or play areas; showering with soap and bathing children before and after going in public pools and recreational areas; and washing hands well after handling diapers.

- Hot tub rash, *pseudomona* folliculitis, is a bacterial colonization of hair follicles in hot, low-pH, improperly chlorinated hot tubs and spas that causes itchy, red bumps and blisters. To avoid this rash, limit time in hot tubs, keep water temperatures below 105 degrees, and properly maintain water chemistry.

- Primary amoebic meningoencephalitis is an uncommon but usually fatal disease from exposure to warm, stagnant waters harboring the amoeba *Naegleri fowleri*. To lower chances of acquiring it, avoid warm, shallow, freshwater ponds and lakes, hot springs, and warm waters near power plants; use a nose clip in lakes and ponds; and don't stir sediment in shallow, warm, freshwater.

- Swimmer's itch, cercarial dermatitis, is an allergic reaction to a parasite in fresh and saltwater that causes skin tingling, burning, or itching, small, reddish pimples, and blisters. The itch can be avoided by staying out of water in marshy areas where the snails that harbor the parasite live and showering and rinsing immediately after exiting the water.

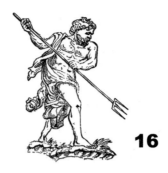

16

Neptune's Revenge
Seafood Allergies

In Mexico we have a word for sushi: bait.

José Simons

Ponce de León may have been looking for fabulous wealth when he stepped ashore in Florida 500 years ago, but it's offshore where the real gold lies today. In 2007, Florida harvested over 82 million pounds of seafood with a dockside value of nearly $175 million. The state boasts more seafood processing plants than any other in the nation and provides more than 200 million seafood dinners annually.[1]

Seafood also turns out to be the most commonly reported food allergy among American adults and potentially one of the most severe, with about 2.5 percent of the population, or about 6.5 million people, allergic to shellfish and finfish, and more than half of sensitive individuals reporting multiple reactions. Up to 15 percent require epinephrine to treat severe reactions.[2] Perhaps not surprisingly, the seafoods at the top of the list in consumption—shrimp and lobster—are also the top allergy triggers, with about 1 in 50 people reporting shellfish allergy.

Mostly an adult-onset allergy, researchers believe the increasing prevalence of seafood allergy is due in large measure to a commensurate increase in seafood consumption (25 percent) since 1970.[3]

Seafood allergy is also more common among women than men and among African Americans (3.7 percent).

And then there's seafood poisoning. But let's look at allergies first.

Fishing for Facts

Seafood allergies basically boil (broil, steam, fry, or grill) down to two types: shellfish allergy and fish allergy. Fish allergy is just what it says: an allergy to scaly, bony fish and sometimes only to certain species. Shellfish allergy, though, goes beyond fish with shells, like the predictable oysters and mussels, collectively known as mollusks (phylum Mollusca, which also includes squid), to include crustaceans (subphylum Crustacea), the hard-bodied delicacies of lobster, crayfish, prawns, crabs, and shrimp. And it's not just as simple as avoiding shrimp scampi or only dining at BBQ joints.

Fish derivatives can end up in dips, spreads, sauces, and garnishes, in gelatin, in ethnic foods, soups, and salad dressings, in fish food, and in cosmetic items like lip balms and glosses, creams, and ointments.[4]

The allergy component in fish is a calcium-binding muscle protein called parvalbumin that is highly cross-reactive between many species of fish.[5] Allergy to cod, one of the most highly consumed fish, is the most commonly reported. Some studies suggest that sensitization to a fish parasite known as *Anisakis simplex*, which can also produce an illness called anisakiasis, may be an allergic trigger.[6] *Anisakis simplex* is also cross-reactive with shrimp and cockroach, suggesting a deeper allergenic connection. Sensitization to *Anisakis simplex* manifests as urticaria or angioedema, even to fish that has been safely cooked.

Some individuals are sensitive only to a particular kind of fish, an allergy most commonly seen with tuna or swordfish. Although if someone experiences an allergic reaction after consuming one type of fish, there may be a 50 percent chance of allergy to at least one other kind of fish. The chance of multiple shellfish allergy is even higher, 75 percent after an initial reaction to shellfish.[7]

Allergic reactions can differ between different species consumed, and although there doesn't seem to be any cross-reaction between shellfish and finfish, the two allergies exist concomitantly.[8] Canned fish products don't seem to provoke allergies to the same extent as fresh fish, suggesting that antigens are affected during processing, and as a matter of fact, allergies to raw fish are more prevalent than allergies to cooked fish.[9]

Occupational asthma is also an issue for those in fish processing industries, and there are plenty of people who handle fish occupationally in Florida, from fishermen to dockhands to restaurant workers. Occupational asthma occurs in up to 36 percent of people professionally handling seafood, triggered by either manual or automated processing of crabs, prawns, mussels, fish, or fishmeal, as well as by cooking vapors and aerosolisation of seafood allergens.

In addition to asthma and other respiratory problems, occupational exposure can result in an allergic skin reaction known as animal protein dermatitis, which affects up to 11 percent of fish industry workers.[10] Animal protein dermatitis can also affect recreational fisherman handling raw bait. And hobby aquarists can suffer "aquarium allergy" from handling fish food, especially chironomid-, daphnia-, and brine shrimp–based foods.

Allergies on the Half Shell

Shrimp is the number one reported shellfish allergy, not surprising since it's relatively inexpensive and, in Florida, available everywhere from roadside vendors to fast food restaurants. Shellfish allergy can also occur with other crustaceans like lobster, prawns and crabs; with bivalves like clams, oysters and scallops; with univalves like conch, limpets, snails and whelks; and with octopus and squid, which are also mollusks.

Tropomyosin, a protein important for muscle contraction in this group, is the principal allergen in shrimp and lobster. Tropomyosin is also a component of dust mite allergen. In one study, an entire population of patients exhibiting snail allergy asthma or rhinitis also suffered from asthma or rhinitis to dust mites. A similar association has been found between shellfish allergy and cockroach allergy.[11]

Shellfish allergy is highly cross-reactive. In one study, 80 percent of patients with shrimp allergy also tested positive for allergies to crab, crayfish, and lobster. A few patients, however, were sensitive only to one particular species of shrimp.[12]

Diagnosing and Treating Seafood Allergy

Allergic reactions to seafood can occur from two to six hours after consuming the trigger food and, in very sensitive individuals, simply from inhaling aerosolized allergens from fish. Symptoms of seafood allergy can include hives and swelling, contact urticaria from handling seafood, gastrointestinal distress, asthma, atopic eczema that worsens after exposure to fish, and seafood-related, exercise induced anaphylaxis (EIA).[13]

Sometimes it's hard to tell whether a bad reaction is allergic in nature, a nonallergic response to something like food poisoning, or a bacterial or viral infection. My husband once had a bad reaction to lobster he ate in New Jersey, not exactly a bastion of fine lobster dining. He swore off lobster for years, convinced he was allergic to it. Not long ago, on a trip to Maine—no visit to which can be complete without at least sampling lobster—he gave it a tentative try and suffered no ill effects.

Then there are people who may not have a bad reaction at all the first time around but aren't as lucky the second time. On the night of their high school prom, Carolyn Lang, of Tampa, and some friends ate at a seaside restaurant in Long Boat Key.

"My friend had eaten swordfish once before," she recalled. So her friend had no reason not to order it for dinner that night. "We left dinner and went to the dance. We walked in, had our pictures taken, and I looked and her entire face was red and swollen. We left and went to the ER. I was at dinner for two hours, prom for 15 minutes, and the ER for five hours. We did make it to the after parties!"

Chances are pretty good that her friend didn't try swordfish a third time.

A proper diagnosis usually consists of skin prick testing, blood tests like the RAST (although the RAST is less effective with shellfish allergy), and a clinical history. Double-blind placebo-controlled food challenges are also a reliable way to assess the extent of a seafood allergy and to narrow down specific problematic species.[14]

Currently, no effective immunotherapy exists for treating seafood allergy, although several studies are under way.[15] The most effective treatment for seafood allergy is to avoid the allergenic food, although it seems many people with seafood allergies can enjoy canned tuna, the least allergenic form of fish.

Atopic children—those whose skin is easily irritated by environmental allergens or foods—should not be given seafood until they are 4, and then starting only with canned tuna. Severely allergic individuals may want to consider wearing a Medic Alert bracelet identifying the extent of the allergy, and they should always carry injectable epinephrine with them.[16]

Having injectable epinephrine might have made all the difference in the world in the 2008 case of a 35-year-old man with shellfish allergy who died of anaphylactic shock at a popular chain restaurant in Georgia. He died within 30 minutes of consuming an entree containing crab. The restaurant said the man never disclosed a seafood allergy. But the entrée was called "Chicken Oscar," and the diner probably never suspected seafood among the ingredients.[17]

Hide and Seek with Seafood

While it may be relatively easy to avoid fish as a stand-alone menu item, avoiding bits of fish and shellfish in the myriad products in which seafood is used is a lot harder. Seafood, it turns out, can occur in an amazing number of items and dishes, including Worcestershire sauce, Caesar salad dressing, caponata, paella, bouillabaisse, fruits de mer, and many Asian dishes. The importance of reading labels and menus and speaking to cooks before ordering or dining can't be overstated.

Health supplements can also pose problems. Although fish protein in fresh fish is the root cause of allergies, fish oil capsules may contain sufficient amounts of fish protein to trigger reactions.[18] Glucosamine supplements, a popular complementary treatment for os-

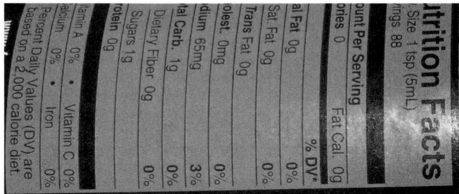

Worcestershire sauce label. (Photo by Theresa Willingham.)

teoarthritis, is made of the exoskeletons of crustaceans, and while that component of shellfish is not allergenic, the product is never guaranteed to be free of protein contaminants, hence the seafood allergy warning on all glucosamine and condroitin products.[19]

Along those lines, cross-contamination is another concern for those with seafood allergy, especially when dining out. Restaurants may use shared equipment, frying chicken where fish has been fried, for instance, or using fish-contaminated utensils on other foods.

Seafood Allergy Myths

One particularly prevalent myth is that someone with seafood allergy is at risk for a reaction if undergoing radioactive imaging that requires ingesting iodine-based contrasts.[20] Seafood allergy is due to sensitivity to seafood proteins, not to their iodine content. Yet the myth persists, in part because the medical community itself propagates it.

One study found that 70 percent of surveyed radiologists and cardiologists regularly asked patients about seafood allergy before administering radio contrast agents, and 40 percent said they wouldn't administer the contrast to patients with seafood allergy. Yet a University of Maryland School of Medicine study concluded that iodine is not an allergen and that the chances of having a reaction to iodine-containing radio contrast agents is the same as it is to any type of contrast—about 0.2–17 percent depending on the contrast—regardless of seafood allergy.[21] "Allergies to shellfish, in particular," researchers E. Schabelman and M. Witting wrote, "do not increase the risk of reaction to intravenous contrast any more that of other allergies."

Another misplaced concern is that those with seafood allergies should avoid carrageenan, a very common food additive used for thickening and stabilizing ingredients in everything from toothpaste to beer to ice cream. Carrageenan is unrelated to fish or shellfish, but it is a type of seaweed and safe for those with seafood allergies to consume.[22]

Other Marine Toxic Illnesses

Because they can sometimes be confused for allergic reactions, but require different treatments, seafood-related toxic illnesses bear mentioning. The most commonly encountered seafood toxic illnesses include scombroid or histamine fish poisoning, nematode *Anisakis simplex*, ciguatera, puffer fish poisoning, and shellfish poisoning.

Scombroid Poisoning

Scombroid poisoning is your basic garden variety food poisoning, a nonallergic, often gastrointestinal reaction to spoiled food. Seafood is the leading cause of food poisoning outbreaks in the United States. Food poisoning due to seafood is usually the result of a type of histamine-related toxin that develops in dark meat fish, typically of the Scombridae and Scomberesocidea families like tuna or mackerel (hence "Scombroid" poisoning), that has spoiled. Other fish, like mahi-mahi, bluefish, and sardines, can also provoke histamine poisoning.[23]

Excessive histamine in the fish develops as bacteria grows, although contaminated fish may not look or smell suspect, nor does cooking destroy the histamine. Reactions are usually mild and can mimic an allergic reaction, producing oral allergy reactions, rashes and hives, itching, and nausea, usually within a few minutes of ingesting contaminated food, and lasting up to 24 hours. Antihistamines can actually be used to effectively treat scombroid poisoning.

Nematode *Anisakis simplex*

Mentioned earlier, reactions to this fish nematode actually are allergic in nature but not considered a seafood allergy per se. Hypersensitivity to *A. simplex* can be a rare cause of anaphylaxis and has been found to provoke rheumatology symptoms. *A. simplex* reactions are most common as a result of consuming raw fish.

Ciguatera

Ciguatera is a type of fish poisoning that can occur from eating large reef fish such as grouper, red snapper, mackerel, or barracuda.[24] It results from eating reef fish that feed on certain dinoflagellates (algae) associated with coral reef systems. The poison stems from ciguatoxins produced by dinoflagellates that have concentrated to toxic levels in the fish's flesh.[25] Cooking or freezing fish does not destroy ciguatoxins, and contaminated fish neither look nor smell bad.

Symptoms can appear within 6 to 24 hours of eating contaminated fish and can include vomiting and diarrhea, abdominal pain, weakness, dizziness, itching, muscle and joint aches, tingling in the hands or feet, or painful urination. A classic symptom of ciguatera is a reversal of temperature sensation: cold things feel or taste hot to the touch, and vice versa.

While rarely fatal, ciguatera is no picnic, and symptoms can recur for weeks or months afterwards. If caught early, within the first couple of days, ciguatera can be treated with Mannitol, an intravenous drug that helps flush ciguatoxins from the system. The risk of ciguatera can be lowered by not consuming large reef fish, especially species like barracuda.

Puffer Fish Poisoning

For some amazing reason, nearly 30 people were diagnosed with puffer fish poisoning in Florida in 2002, resulting in the need for the Florida Fish and Wildlife Conservation Commission to issue a ban on eating Florida puffer fish in Volusia, Brevard, North Indian River, Martin and St. Lucie counties.[26] Anyone who has seen a puffer fish may wonder why someone would eat one in the first place, but they're considered something of a delicacy in some cultures.

As if their armored, inflationary self-defense mechanism weren't enough to discourage predation, puffer fish also harbor something called tetrodotoxin in their skin and organs as well as saxitoxin in their flesh. Symptoms of puffer fish poisoning can occur within minutes and include numbness and tingling of the face and extremities,

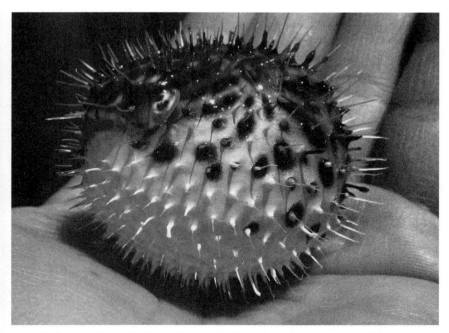

Puffer fish. (Photo by Bruce Moravchik, "Islands in the Stream Expedition 2002," Office of Ocean Exploration and Research, courtesy of NOAA/USDC.)

muscle weakness, and nausea and vomiting. The best defense here is
a good offense: Don't eat puffer fish!

Shellfish Poisoning

The most common type of shellfish poisoning in Florida is neurotoxic shellfish poisoning (NSP), discussed in the previous chapter.
Caused by the dinoflagellate that produces red tide, NSP develops
within one to three hours of eating contaminated shellfish. Symptoms include numbness, tingling of the mouth, arms, and legs, poor
coordination, and sometimes temperature reversal. Recovery typically occurs within a couple of days without any intervention. Shellfish poisoning is best avoided by not eating local shellfish during
periods of red tide bloom.

So there you have it, a dozen ways to Sunday to get sick on seafood. As with most things, though, if common sense prevails—read
menus and labels thoroughly if you have an allergy, eat fresh fish
from reliable suppliers and known sources, and don't eat fish that
make it clear they shouldn't be eaten—you're far more likely to stay
healthy than not.

In Summary

- Seafood is the most commonly reported food allergy among
  American adults, affecting about 2.5 percent of the population, or about 6.5 million people.
- Seafood allergies are of two types: allergy to shellfish, typically shrimp, and allergy to fish, typically cod.
- An allergic reaction to one type of fish increases likelihood
  of allergic reaction to at least one other kind of fish by 50
  percent. The likelihood of allergy to multiple shellfish is even
  higher—75 percent after an initial reaction to one kind.
- Canned fish products are less allergenic than fresh fish, and
  allergies to raw fish are more prevalent than allergies to
  cooked fish.
- Occupational asthma occurs in up to 36 percent of people

who handle seafood professionally, and 11 percent of industry workers can experience animal protein dermatitis.

- Shellfish allergy is highly cross-reactive within the shellfish family as well as to dust mite and cockroach allergens.
- Seafood allergy is usually diagnosed by skin prick testing, through blood tests like the RAST, and with reference to a sufferer's clinical history. The most effective tests are double-blind placebo-controlled food challenges.
- Currently, no effective immunotherapy exists for treating seafood allergy, although several are under study. Prevention by avoidance of trigger seafood is the best practice.
- Because severe seafood allergy can result in anaphylaxis, highly allergic individuals should always carry injectable epinephrine with them; they might also consider wearing a Medic Alert bracelet that identifies the type and severity of allergy.
- Hidden seafood occurs in many different food items including sauces and salad dressings, so label reading is important. Cross-contamination is also a consideration when dining out.
- Seafood allergy does not increase the risk of a reaction to iodine-based radioactive contrasts used in medical tests. Iodine is extremely rare and is not related to seafood allergy.
- People with seafood allergies can safely consume products with carrageenan, a seaweed rather than a seafood.
- Other marine toxins that may mimic seafood allergy include scombroid fish poisoning, *Anisakis simplex*, ciguatera, and shellfish poisoning.

In the End

There's obviously a lot more to Florida than meets the eye. From its midge-infested sugar sand beaches to its poison-ivy-laced hardwood hammocks, from its pollen-laden sand-pine scrub and its hives-inducing citrus groves to its eye-watering red-tide-tinged reef waters teeming with allergenic seafood, there's plenty here to get under your skin. Simply put, Florida bites.

But nearly 20 million residents clearly aren't bothered enough to leave, nor are 85 million tourists a year discouraged from visiting. The fact is, for the most part antihistamines keep hay fever at bay, bug spray is effective, and it's easy enough to avoid poison ivy and allergenic foods. Most of the time Florida is a paradise on earth, a spectacular place of unparalleled beauty with endless recreational opportunities for relaxation, exercise, and more.

Knowing where the dangers and discomforts lie and how they make us itch, scratch, sneeze, and otherwise wreak havoc on our human systems can help empower us to safely coexist with the living things in our supra-organic Eden and to better appreciate their beauty and complexity. Respecting the wildness we can only marginally tame frees us to live as part of this beautiful state, in full enjoyment of all the gifts it offers us.

Notes

Introduction: *Gesundheit!* Welcome to Florida

1. Teresa Divers, Jim Farr, Carrie Hall, Jill Huntington, Kim Mikita, and Heidi Recksiek, *Florida Assessment of Coastal Trends 2000,* Florida Department of Community Affairs, Tallahassee, http://www.dep.state.fl.us/cmp/publications/FACT2000.pdf.

2. J. H. Frank and E. D. McCoy, "Precinctive Insect Species in Florida," *Florida Entomologist Online* 78, no. 1 (1995), http://www.fcla.edu/FlaEnt/fe78p21.pdf.

3. Richard P. Wunderlin, *Atlas of Florida Vascular Plants,* 2008, http://www.plantatlas.usf.edu/about.asp.

4. *U.S. Census State and County Quick Facts: Florida* (Washington: Government Printing Office, 2009).

5. Florida Fish and Wildlife Commission, *FWC Fast Facts,* March 2009.

6. David Cheng, "Jellyfish Stings," www.emedicinehealth.com/jellyfish_stings/article_em.htm.

7. *Palynology at the Florida Museum of Natural History,* 13 October 2008, http://www.flmnh.ufl.edu/pollen.htm.

8. American Academy of Allergy, Asthma & Immunology, "Allergy Statistics," http://www.aaaai.org/media/resources/media_kit/allergy_statistics.stm.

9. Alfred I. Neugut, "Anaphylaxis in the United States," *Archives of Internal Medicine* 161 (8 January 2001): 15–21.

10. "Tips to Remember: Allergic Reactions" *Patients and Consumers,* 2008, http://www.aaaai.org/patients/publicedmat/tips/whatisallergicreaction.stm.

Part I. Florida Seasons: Hay Fever Season, Mold Season, Oak Pollen Season

1. Thomas Leo Ogren, *Allergy-Free Gardening: The Revolutionary Guide to Healthy Landscaping* (Berkeley: Ten Speed Press, 2000).
2. Thomas Leo Ogren, *Safe Sex in the Garden: And Other Propositions for an Allergy-Free World* (Berkeley: Ten Speed Press, 2003).
3. John H. Krouse, Stephen J. Chadwick, Bruce R. Gordon, and M. Jennifer Derebery, *Allergy and Immunology: An Otolaryngic Approach* (Philadelphia: Lippincott Williams & Wilkins, 2002).

Chapter 1. Happy New Year! It's Tree Pollen Season

1. Mary L. Jelks, "Florida Pollen Review," *Allergy and Asthma Proceedings* 11, no. 6 (November/December 1990): 273–80.
2. Nancy P. Arny, *Common Oaks of Florida*, Fact Sheet FOR 51, School of Forest Resources and Conservation, Florida Cooperative Extension Service, Institute of Food and Agricultural Sciences, University of Florida (hereafter UF/IFAS Extension), June 1996, http://edis.ifas.ufl.edu/fr004.
3. "AAAAI: Oral Allergy Syndrome Made Worse by Ragweed, Fruits, and Vegetables," *RedOrbit*, 15 August 2007, http://www.redorbit.com/news/health/1034373/aaaai_oral_allergy_syndrome_made_worse_by_ragweed_fruits_and/index.html.
4. Linda Conway Duever, "*Casuarina equisetifolia*," *Floridata*, 18 June 2004, http://www.floridata.com/ref/c/casu_equ.cfm.
5. Harris Steinman, "Australian Pine," Phadia, 2008, http://www.phadia.com/en/Allergen-information/ImmunoCAP-Allergens/Tree-Pollens/Allergens/Australian-pine.
6. Ogren, *Allergy-Free Gardening*.
7. Daniel Culbert, *Red, White, and Black Mulberries for Florida Yards*, UF/IFAS Okeechobee County Extension Service, 11 April 2006, http://okeechobee.ifas.ufl.edu/News.columns/Mulberries.for.Florida.Yards.htm; Harris Steinman, "Red Mulberry," http://www.phadia.com/en/Allergen-information/ImmunoCAP-Allergens/Tree-Pollens/Allergens/Red-mulberry/.
8. USDA-ARS Invasive Plant Research Laboratory, *A Century of Melaleuca Invasion in South Florida*, brochure, Ft. Lauderdale, 2004.
9. Harris Steinman, "Melaleuca," Phadia, 2008 http://www.phadia.com/en/Allergen-information/ImmunoCAP-Allergens/Tree-Pollens/Allergens/Melaleuca-Cajeput-tree/.
10. National Institute of Environmental Health Sciences (NIEHS), "Pollen," http://www.niehs.nih.gov.
11. Ed Perratore, "California Regulates 'Ozone Generator' Air Purifiers," *Consumer Reports*, 15 October 2007.

Chapter 2. Springtime in Paradise

1. C. Milesi, S. W. Running, C. D. Elvidge, J. B. Dietz, B. T. Tuttle, and R. R. Nemani, "Mapping and Modeling the Biogeochemical Cycling of Turf Grasses in the United States," *Environmental Management* 36, no. 3 (2005): 426–38.

2. J. J. Haydu, L. N. Satterthwaite, and J. L. Cisar, "An Economic and Agronomic Profile of Florida's Sod Industry in 2003," http://edis.ifas.ufl.edu/pdffiles/FE/FE56100.pdf.

3. "More Than Half the U.S. Population Is Sensitive to One or More Allergens," *National Institutes of Health News*, 4 August 2005, http://www.nih.gov/news/pr/aug2005/niehs-04.htm.

4. "Grass Biology," *Grasses of Palm Beach and Martin Counties*, http://floridagrasses.org/Grass%20Biology.htm.

5. John H. Krouse, M. Jennifer Derebery, and Stephen J. Chadwick, *Managing the Allergic Patient* (Philadelphia: Saunders Elsevier, 2007), 24–25.

6. Ibid.

7. Jim Conrad, "Grass Flowers," http://www.backyardnature.net/fl_grass.htm.

8. Samuel J. Arbes Jr., Peter J. Gergen, Leslie Elliott, and Darryl C. Zeldin, "Prevalences of Positive Skin Test Responses to 10 Common Allergens in the U.S. Population: Results from the Third National Health and Nutrition Examination Survey," *Journal of Allergy and Clinical Immunology* 116, no. 2 (August 2005): 377–83.

9. Richard L. Duble, *Bermudagrass: The Sports Turf of the South*, http://aggie-horticulture.tamu.edu/archives/parsons/turf/publications/bermuda.html.

10. Frances Northall, "Vegetation, Vegetables, Vesicles: Plants and Skin," http://www.redorbit.com/news/science/17674/vegetation_vegetables_vesicles_plants_and_skin/.

11. "Oral Allergy Syndrome," http://allergies.about.com/od/foodallergies/a/oas.htm.http

12. Thomas Leo Ogren, "The Pollen-Trapping Power of a Lawn," http://www.american-lawns.com/pollen.html.

13. K. Ivory, S. J. Chambers, C. Pin, E. Prieto, J. L. Arqués, and C. Nicoletti, "Oral Delivery of *Lactobacillus casei* Shirota Modifies Allergen-Induced Immune Responses in Allergic Rhinitis," *Clinical & Experimental Allergy* 38, no. 8 (August 2008): 1282–89.

14. L. Frølund, S. R. Durham, M. Calderon, W. Emminger, J. S. Andersen, P. Rask, and R. Dahl, "Sustained Effect of SQ-Standardized Grass Allergy Immunotherapy Tablet on Rhinoconjunctivitis Quality of Life," *Allergy* 65, no. 6 (2010): 753–57.

Chapter 3. Ragweed, the Scourge of Summer and Fall

1. Estelle Levetin, "Ragweed," http://pollen.utulsa.edu/ragweed.htm.

2. Matthew Josephson, "Edison: Last Days of the Wizard," *American Heritage* 10, no. 6 (1959).

3. M. S. Hawkins, "Goldenrod," *Complimentary Medicine*, 17 January 2007, http://www.umm.edu/altmed/articles/goldenrod-000251.htm.

4. Dan Culbert, "Falling for Yellow Wildflowers," 23 October 2005, http://okeechobee.ifas.ufl.edu/News%20columns/Fall%20Yellow%20Wildflowers.htm.

5. Daniel E. Moerman, *Native American Ethnobotany* (Portland, Ore.: Timber Press, 1998), 66.

6. "Ragweed Allergy," *Allergies,* 2005, http://www.aafa.org.

7. Levetin, "Ragweed."

8. "Ragweed Allergy."

9. Anthony Ham Pong, "Oral Allergy Syndrome," http://www.calgaryallergy.ca/Articles/English/Oral_Food_Allergy.htm.

10. "Ragweed Allergy," Asthma and Allergy Foundation of America, 2005, http://www.aafa.org/display.cfm?id=9&sub=24&cont=349.

11. "Experimental Ragweed Therapy Offers Allergy Sufferers Longer Relief with Fewer Shots," *National Institutes of Health News*, 4 October 2006, http://www.nih.gov/news/pr/oct2006/niaid-04.htm.

12. Charlene Laino, "Fight Ragweed Allergies without Shots: Placing Allergen Extract under the Tongue May Reduce Need for Antihistamines," *WebMD Health News*, 19 March 2008, http://www.webmd.com/allergies/news/20080319/fighting-ragweed-allergies-sans-shots.

Chapter 4. A Fungus Among Us

1. D. L. Hawksworth, "The Magnitude of Fungal Diversity: The 1.5 Million Species Estimate Revisited," *Mycological Research* 105, no. 12 (2001): 1422–32.

2. Laurence B. Molloy, "Pathogenic Fungi," *Molloy Environmental,* 1999, http://users.rcn.com/leadsafe/fungi.html.

3. "News from the ACAAI: Experts Sort Fact from Fiction on Health Effects of Mold," 5 November 2005, http://myallergyasthma.com/images/health_effects_of_mold.pdf.

4. Barzin Khalili, Marc T. Montanaro, and Emil J. Bardana Jr., "Indoor Mold and Your Patient's Health: From Suspicion to Confirmation," *Journal of Respiratory Diseases* 5, no. 12 (December 2005).

5. Committee on Environmental Health, "Toxic Effects of Indoor Molds," *Pediatrics* 101, no. 4 (4 April 1998): 712–14, http://aappolicy.aappublications.org/cgi/content/full/pediatrics;101/4/712.

6. Molloy, "Pathogenic Fungi."

7. Ibid.; Clyde M. Christensen. *The Molds and Man,* 3rd ed. (Minneapolis: University of Minnesota Press, 1965).

8. Wallace Ravven, "One of Life's Most Common Compounds Causes Allergic Inflammation," *ICSF Today*, 23 April 1997, http://pub.ucsf.edu/today/cache/feature/200704205.html.

9. "Experts Sort Fact from Fiction on Health Effects of Mold," *Public Education,*

American College of Allergy, Asthma & Immunology, 9 November 2005, http://www.acaai.org/public/NR/Fungal.htm.

10. Jay Portnoy, Susan Flappan, and Charles S. Barnes, "A Procedure for Evaluation of the Indoor Environment," *Aerobiologia* 17, no. 1 (March 2001): 43–48.

11. Robert J. Black, "Florida Climate Data," UF/IFAS, July 1993, http://edis.ifas.ufl.edu/eh105.

12. Florida Solar Energy Center, "Humidity," 2007, http://www.fsec.ucf.edu/en/consumer/buildings/basics/humidity.htm.

13. Editorial Board, "Mold Allergy," Asthma and Allergy Foundation of America (AAFA), 2005, http://www.aafa.org/print.cfm?id=8&sub=16&cont=58.

Part II. What's Bugging You?

1. J. H. Frank and E. D. McCoy, "Precinctive Insect Species in Florida," *Florida Entomologist* 78, no. 1 (1995): 21–35.

2. Department of Systematic Biology, "Numbers of Insects (Species and Individuals)," *Bug Info*, Smithsonian Institute, http://www.si.edu/encyclopedia_si/nmnh/buginfo/bugnos.htm.

3. P. G. Koehler and F. M. Oi, *Stinging or Venomous Insects and Related Pests*, UF/IFAS Extension, Pub. ENY-215, June 2007, http://edis.ifas.ufl.edu/IG099.

4. Ibid.

5. American Academy of Allergy, Asthma, and Immunology, *Stinging Insect Allergy*, 2009, http://www.aaaai.org/patients/virtual_allergist/insect.asp.

6. Philip Koehler, "Dealing with Yellowjackets," 2 October 1998, http://entnemdept.ufl.edu/PestAlert/pgk-1002.htm.

7. Peter C. Schalock, "Dermatitis," *Merck Manuals Online Medical Library*, December 2006, http://www.merck.com/mmhe/sec18/ch203/ch203c.html.

Chapter 5. Beeware of Hymenoptera, Part I: Bees and Wasps

1. Josh Zimmer and Tamara Lush, "Yellow Jackets Swarm, Kill Man," *St. Petersburg Times*, 16 April 2002, http://www.sptimes.com/2002/04/16/TampaBay/Yellow_jackets_swarm_.shtml.

2. "AAAI Offers Advice on Stinging Insect Allergies," *Health Education Library for People*, 6 June 2007, http://www.healthlibrary.com/news378.htm.

3. P. G. Koehler and F. M. Oi, *Stinging or Venomous Insects and Related Pests*, UF/IFAS Extension, Pub. ENY-215, June 2007, http://edis.ifas.ufl.edu/IG099.

4. Mark Deyrup and Thomas C. Emmel, *Florida's Fabulous Insects* (Hawaiian Gardens, Calif.: World Publications, 2000).

5. J. Fernandez, M. Blanca, V. Soriano, J. Sanchez, and C. Juarez, "Epidemiological Study of the Prevalence of Allergic Reactions to Hymenoptera in Rural Populations in the Mediterranean Area," *Clinical and Experimental Allergy* 29, no. 8 (August 1999): 1069–74.

6. Malcolm Sanford, "Bee Stings and 'Allergic' Reactions," UF/IFAS Extension, 1 May 2003, http://edis.ifas.ufl.edu/aa159.

7. Howard S. Rubenstein, "Bee-Sting Diseases," *Lancet* 319 (27 February 1982): 496–99.

8. S. O. Stapel, J. Waanders-Lijster de Raadt, A. W. van Toorenenbergen, and H. de Groot, "Allergy to Bumblebee Venom. II. IgE Cross-Reactivity between Bumblebee and Honeybee Venom," *Allergy* 53, no. 8 (August 1998): 769–77.

9. A. Kettner, H. Henry, G. Hyghes, G. Corradin, and F. Spertini, "IgE and T-cell Responses to High-Molecular Weight Allergens from Bee Venom," *Clinical and Experimental Allergy* 29, no. 3 (March 1999): 394–401.

10. Beatriz Moisset, "Anthophila (Apoidea)—Bees," *Bug Guide*, Iowa State University Entomology Department, 27 October 2004, http://bugguide.net/node/view/8267.

11. John B. Pascarella, "The Bees of Florida," 23 September 2008, http://www.bio.georgiasouthern.edu/Bio-home/Pascarella/Intro.htm.

12. Deyrup and Emmel, *Florida's Fabulous Insects.*

13. Everett Oertel, "History of Beekeeping in the United States," *Beesource*, Agriculture Handbook 335, October 1980, http://www.beesource.com/resources/usda/history-of-beekeeping-in-the-united-states/.

14. James D. Ellis and Amanda Ellis, *African Honey Bee, Africanized Honey Bee, Killer Bee,* Apis mellifera scutellata *Lepeletier (Insecta: Hymenoptera: Apidea),* UF/IFAS Extension, Pub. EENY 429, November 2009, edis.ifas.ufl.edu/pdffiles/IN/IN79000.pdf.

15. P. Kirk Visscher, Richard S. Vetter, and Scott Camazine, *Removing Bee Stings: Speed Matters, Method Doesn't,* 1996, http://bees.ucr.edu/stings.html.

16. David B. K. Golden, "Insect Sting Allergy and Venom Immunotherapy: A Model and a Mystery," *Journal of Allergy and Clinical Immunology* 115, no. 3 (March 2005): 439–47.

17. Philip G. Koehler, Donald E. Short, and William H. Kern Jr., *Pests in and around the Florida Home,* 3rd ed. (Gainesville: Florida Cooperative Extension Service, 1995), 63.

18. Ibid.

19. Pamela W. Ewan, "ABC of Allergies: Venom Allergy," *British Medical Journal* 316 (2 May 1998): 1365–68.

20. West Virginia University Extension Service, *About Bee and Wasp Stings,* February 1998, http://www.wvu.edu/~agexten/wildlife/bees.htm.

21. Lionel A. Stange, "Cicada Killer, Giant Ground Hornet," *Featured Creatures,* UF/IFAS Extension, July 2009, http://entnemdept.ufl.edu/creatures/beneficial/cicada_killers.htm.

22. John Foltz, "Hymenoptera: Ichneumonoidea: Ichneumonidae," *ENY 3005 Family Identification,* University of Florida Department of Entomology and Nematology, 12 June 2001, http://entomology.ifas.ufl.edu/foltz/eny3005/lab1/Hymenoptera/Ichneumonid.htm.

23. Deyrup and Emmel, *Florida's Fabulous Insects.*

24. E. E. Grissell and Thomas R. Fasulo, "Yellowjackets and Hornets," *Featured Creatures,* UF/IFAS Extension, August 2010, http://entnemdept.ufl.edu/creatures/urban/occas/hornet_yellowjacket.htm.

25. Gordon Ramel, "The Social Wasps (*Vespidae*)," *Earth Life Web,* 19 May 2009, http://www.earthlife.net/insects/socwasps.html#Polistine.

26. "Largest Yellow Jacket Nest Ever Documented?" *WALB News 10 Update,* 28 June 2006, http://www.walb.com/Global/story.asp?S=5092001&clienttype=printable.

27. "Bee Remover: Biggest Yellow Jacket Nest Ever in City," WFTV 9, 21 June 2006, http://www.wftv.com/news/9406678/detail.html.

28. Koehler et al., *Pests in and around the Florida Home.*

Chapter 6. Hymenoptera, Part II: The Ants

1. T. M. Freeman, "Hymenoptera Hypersensitivity in an Imported Fire Ant Endemic Area," *Annals of Allergy, Asthma, and Immunology* 78 (1997): 369–72.

2. Emma Willcox and William M. Giuliano, "Red Imported Fire Ants and Their Impacts on Wildlife," Department of Wildlife Ecology and Conservation, UF/IFAS Extension, April 2006.

3. Laura Collins and Rudolf H. Scheffrahn, "Red Imported Fire Ant: Solenopsis invicta Buren (Insecta: Hymenoptera: Formicidae: Myrmicinae)," *Featured Creatures,* August 2008, UF/IFAS Extension, http://entnem.ufl.edu/creatures/urban/ants/red_imported_fire_ant.htm.

4. Lewis R. Goldfrank, Neal E. Flomenbaum, and Lewis S. Nelson, *Goldfrank's Toxicologic Emergencies,* 7th ed. (New York: McGraw-Hill Medical, 2002).

5. D. R. Hoffman, "Fire and Venom Allergy," *Allergy* 50 (1995): 535–44.

6. Willcox and Giuliano, "Red Imported Fire Ants."

7. Collins and Scheffrahn, "Red Imported Fire Ant."

8. Mark Deyrup and Thomas C. Emmel, *Florida's Fabulous Insects* (Hawaiian Gardens, Calif.: World Publications, 2000), 167.

9. J. H. Klotz et al., "Adverse Reactions to Ants Other than Imported Fire Ants," *Annals of Allergy, Asthma, and Immunology* 95 (2005): 418–25.

10. Shawn Brooks and J. C. Nickerson, "Little Fire Ant, Wasmannia auropunctata," UF/IFAS Extension, March 2008, http://edis.ifas.ufl.edu/IN296.

11. Deyrup and Emmel, *Florida's Fabulous Insects.*

12. Collins and Schreffahn, "Red Imported Fire Ant."

13. Patricia Toth, "Elongate Twig Ant, Mexican Twig Ant: Pseudomyrmex gracilis (Insecta: Hymenoptera: Formicidae: Myrmicinae)," *Featured Creatures,* UF/IFAS Extension, September 2007, http://entnemdept.ufl.edu/creatures/misc/ants/elongate_twig_ant.htm.

14. Deyrup and Emmel, *Florida's Fabulous Insects.*

15. T. J. Walker, *University of Florida Book of Insect Records,* 2001, chap. 23, http://entomology.ifas.ufl.edu/walker/ufbir/.

16. Deyrup and Emmel, *Florida's Fabulous Insects.*

17. J. C. Nickerson, "Florida Harvester Ant: Pogonomyrmex badius (Latreille) (Insecta: Hymenoptera: Formicidae)," *Featured Creatures,* UF/IFAS Extension, June 2003, http://entnem.ufl.edu/creatures/urban/ants/harvester_ant.htm.

18. D. L. Wray, "Notes on the Southern Harvester Ant (Pogonomyrmex badius Latr.) in North Carolina," *Annals of the Entomological Society of America* 31 (1938): 196–201.

19. K. D. Haack and T. A. Granovsky, "Ants," in *Handbook of Pest Control,* ed. K. Story and D. Moreland (Cleveland: Franzak & Foster, 1990), 415–79.

20. John Warner and Rudolf H. Scheffrahn, "Florida Carpenter Ant, Bull Ant, Tortugas Carpenter Ant, Camponotus floridanus (Buckley), and Camponotus tortuganus (Emery) (Insecta: Hymenoptera: Formicidae: Subfamily ormicinae: Tribe Camponotini)," *EDIS,* March 2008, http://edis.ifas.ufl.edu/IN455.

21. James Ralston, MD, "Fire Ant Bites: Treatment and Medication," November 2009, http://emedicine.medscape.com/article/1089027-treatment.

22. William Boggs, MD, "Rush Immunotherapy Protocol for Imported Fire Ants Safe for Young Children," *Reuters Health Information,* September 2008, http://www.medscape.com/viewarticle/581230_print.

23. Philip G. Koehler, Donald E. Short, and William H. Kern Jr., *Pests in and around the Florida Home,* Florida Cooperative Extension Service, 3rd ed., 1995.

24. Collins and Scheffrahn, "Red Imported Fire Ant."

25. Koehler and Short, *Pests in and around the Florida Home.*

26. William Vitka, "Nursing Home Ant-Bite Death Payout: Kin of Patient Killed by Ant Attack Get Nearly $2 Million," *CBS News,* 12 March 2005, http://www.cbsnews.com/stories/2005/03/12/health/main679757.shtml.

27. J. Goddard, J. Jarratt, and R. D. deShazo, "Recommendations for Prevention and Management of Fire Ant Infestation of Health Care Facilities," *Southern Medical Journal* 95, no. 6 (June 2002): 627–33.

28. Larry Gilbert, "Fire Ants, Armadillos, and Phorid Flies—Answers to Frequently Asked Questions," *sciLINKS,* University of Texas at Austin, 17 December 2004,http://uts.cc.utexas.edu/~gilbert/research/fireants/faqans.html.

29. "Pest Control: Ants Become Headless Zombies," MSNBC, 13 May 2009, http://www.msnbc.msn.com/id/30729694/.

30. Goddard et al., "Recommendations for Prevention and Management."

31. Koehler and Short, *Pests in and around the Florida Home.*

32. J. Goddard, "Personal Protection Measures against Fire Ant Attacks," *Annals of Allergy, Asthma & Immunology* 95, no. 4 (October 2005): 344–49.

33. Gilbert, "Fire Ants, Armadillos, and Phorid Flies."

Chapter 7. La Cucaracha

1. Richard Cohn, Samuel J. Arbes Jr., Renee Jaramillo, Laura H. Reid, and Darryl C. Zeldin, "National Prevalence and Exposure Risk for Cockroach Allergen in U.S.

Households," *Medscape Today,* Environmental Health Perspectives, 27 April 2006, http://www.medscape.com/viewarticle/530464_2.

2. Richard F. Lockey, Samuel C. Bukantz, and Jean Bousquet, eds., *Allergens and Allergen Immunotherapy,* 3rd ed. (New York: Marcel Dekker, 2004).

3. "NIAID Study: Cockroaches Important Cause of Asthma Morbidity among Inner-City Children," *NIH News,* National Institute of Allergy and Infectious Diseases (NIAID), 7 May 1997, http://www.nih.gov/news/pr/may97/niaid-7a.htm.

4. Asthma and Allergy Foundation of America (AAFA), "Cockroach Allergy," 2005, http://www.aafa.org/display.cfm?id=9&sub=22&cont=312.

5. P. A. Eggleston and L. K. Arruda, "Ecology and Elimination of Cockroaches and Allergens in the Home," *Journal of Allergy and Clinical Immunology* 107, no. 3 (2001): S422–29.

6. Lockey et al., *Allergens and Allergen Immunotherapy,* 86.

7. National Prevalence and Exposure Risk for Cockroach Allergen, 1997, http://www.medscape.com/viewarticle/530464_4.

8. AAFA, "Cockroach Allergy."

9. P. G. Koehler, F. M. Oi and D. Branscome, *Cockroaches and Their Management,* UF/IFAS Extension, Pub. ENY-214, 2009, http://edis.ifas.ufl.edu/ig082.

10. Mark Deyrup and Thomas C. Emmel, *Florida's Fabulous Insects* (Hawaiian Gardens, Calif.: World Publications, 2000).

11. Philip G. Koehler and Donald E. Short, *Pests in and around the Florida Home,* 2d ed., Florida Cooperative Extension Service, 1995.

12. Barbara Kathryn, "Common Name: American Cockroach," *Featured Creature,* UF/IFAS Extension, 2008, http://entnemdept.ufl.edu/creatures/urban/roaches/american_cockroach.htm.

13. Eggleston and Arruda, "Ecology and Elimination of Cockroaches."

14. Koehler and Short, *Pests in and around the Florida Home.*

15. Mickey Anderson, "UF Entomologists Warn Floridians New Roaches May Be on the Way," *IFAS News,* UF/IFAS Extension, 8 October 2008, http://news.ifas.ufl.edu/2008/10/08/uf-entomologists-warn-floridians-new-roaches-may-be-on-the-way/.

16. Lockey et al., *Allergens and Allergen Immunotherapy,* 194.

17. "Sublingual Cockroach Safety Study (SCSS)," *Clinical Trials,* National Institute of Allergy and Infectious Diseases (NIAID), 12 February 2007, http://clinical-trials.gov/ct2/show/NCT00434421?term=Allergy&recr=Open&rank=31.

Chapter 8. Along Came an Arachnid

1. J. J. Sacks, M. Kresnow, and B. Houston, "Dog Bites: How Big a Problem?" *Injury Prevention* 2 (1996): 52–54; H. B. Weiss, D. Friedman, and J. H. Coben, "Incidence of Dog Bite Injuries Treated in Emergency Departments," *Journal of the American Medical Association* 279 (1998): 51–53; Clay Harris, "Spider Bites," Ohio

State University, 28 March 2009, http://www.marion.ohio-state.edu/SpiderWeb/Spider%20Bites.htm.

2. Harris, "Spider Bites."

3. Terry Thormin, "Potentially Medically Significant Spiders of North America," *Invertebrate Zoology: Research & Projects,* Royal Alberta Museum, 28 March 2009, http://www.royalalbertamuseum.ca/natural/insects/research/dangspid.htm.

4. Roger Highfield, "Spider Venom Could Be Used in Impotence Treatment," *Telegraph,* 16 September 2008, http://www.telegraph.co.uk/scienceandtechnology/science/sciencenews/3351887/Spider-venom-could-be-used-in-impotence-treatment.html.

5. G. B. Edwards and Sam Marshall, *Florida's Fabulous Spiders* (Hawaiian Gardens, Calif.: World Publications, 2002).

6. California Poison Control System, "Spider Bites," 2008, http://www.calpoison.org/public/spiders.html.

7. G. K. Isbister and M. R. Gray. "A Prospective Study of 750 Definite Spider Bites, with Expert Spider Identification," *QJM: An International Journal of Medicine* 95 (2002): 723–31.

8. Edwards and Marshall, *Florida's Fabulous Spiders.*

9. Sean P. Bush, MD, and Jennifer C. Smith, MD, "Spider Envenomation, Widow," *eMedicine,* 24 July 2008, http://emedicine.medscape.com/article/772196-overview.

10. Edwards and Marshall, *Florida's Fabulous Spiders.*

11. G. B. Edwards, "Brown Recluse Spider," *Featured Creatures,* June 2009, UF/IFAS Extension, July 2009, http://entnemdept.ufl.edu/creatures/urban/spiders/brown_recluse_spider.htm.

12. Edwards and Marshall, *Florida's Fabulous Spiders.*

13. G. B. Edwards and K. L. Hibbard, "Mexican Redrump Tarantula," *Featured Creatures,* UF/IFAS Extension, May 2003, http://entomology.ifas.ufl.edu/creatures/misc/spiders/M_redrump.htm.

14. Eric T. Schreiber, "Florida Spiders: Biology and Control," *EntGuide 7,* Public Health Entomology Research and Education Center, 26 October 2006, http://www.pherec.org/EntGuides/EntGuide7.pdf.

15. Ibid.

16. Jerry R. Balentine, DO, FACEP, "Black Widow Spider Bite," *eMedicine-Health,* May 2008, http://www.emedicinehealth.com/black_widow_spider_bite/page11_em.htm.

17. Richard S. Vetter and Sean P. Bush, "Reports of Presumptive Brown Recluse Spider Bites Reinforce Improbable Diagnosis in Regions of North America Where the Spider Is Not Endemic," *Clinical Infectious Diseases* 35, no. 4 (2002): 442–45.

18. Schreiber, "Florida Spiders."

19. Dan Culbert, "Florida Scorpions," UF/IFAS Okeechobee County Extension Service, 10 April 2005, http://okeechobee.ifas.ufl.edu/News%20columns/Florida.Scorpions.htm.

20. Richard Vetter and P. Kirk Visscher, "Bites and Stings of Medically Important Venomous Arthropods," *Entomology—Spiders,* University of California Riverside, 1998, http://spiders.ucr.edu/dermatol.html.

21. J. S. Nugent, D. R. More, L. L. Hagan, J. G. Demain, B. A. Whisman, and T. M. Freeman, "Cross-Reactivity between Allergens in the Venom of the Common Striped Scorpion and the Imported Fire Ant," *Journal of Allergy and Clinical Immunology* 114, no. 2 (August 2004): 383–86; Andy Nish, "Venom Allergy," *Allergy & Asthma Advocate,* American Academy of Allergy Asthma & Immunology, 2007, http://www.aaaai.org/patients/advocate/2007/summer/venom.asp.

22. Culbert, "Florida Scorpions."

23. "Scorpion Stings," Mayo Clinic, 22 November 2008, http://www.mayoclinic.com/health/scorpion-stings/DS01113/DSECTION=prevention.

24. David Evans Walter, Gerald Krantz, and Evert Lindquist, "Acari: The Mites," Tree of Life Project, December 1996, http://tolweb.org/Acari/2554/1996.12.13.

25. Jason Pike, "Blood-Sucking Behavior and Saliva of Blood-Sucking Insects," Colorado State University, 2001, http://www.colostate.edu/Depts/Entomology/courses/en507/papers_2001/pike.htm.

26. P. G. Koehler, "Mites That Attack Humans," UF/IFAS Extension, April 2003, http://edis.ifas.ufl.edu/IG086.

27. Beth Massey, "Straw Itch Mite," West Virginia University Extension Service. July 2000, http://www.wvu.edu/~agexten/ipm/insects/strawmit.htm.

28. Koehler, "Mites That Attack Humans."

29. F. Carswell, "State of the Art: Mites and Human Allergy," *Immunology* 65, no. 4 (December 1988): 497–500.

30. Emily T. Chu, MD, and Alan B. Goldsobel, MD, "House Dust Mite, Cat, and Cockroach Allergen Concentrations in Day Care Centers in Tampa, Florida," *Pediatrics* 110 (August 2002): 430–31.

31. Koehler, "Mites That Attack Humans."

32. William F. Lyon, "House Dust Mites," *Ohio State University Extension Fact Sheet,* http://ohioline.osu.edu/hyg-fact/2000/2157.html.

33. P. G. Koehler and F. M. Oi, "Chiggers," UF/IFAS Extension, February 2003, http://edis.ifas.ufl.edu/IG085.

34. James E. Cilek and Eric T. Schreiber, "Biology and Control of Chiggers," *Ent-Guide 6,* Public Health Entomology Research & Education Center, http://pherec.org/EntGuides/EntGuide6.pdf

35. Ibid.

36. Phillip Hamman, "Chiggers," *House and Landscape Pests,* Texas Agricultural Extension Service, 10 July 2002, http://insects.tamu.edu/extension/bulletins/L-1223.html.

37. Florida Department of Health, Tallahassee, "Rocky Mountain Spotted Fever," http://www.doh.state.fl.us/environment/medicine/arboviral/Tick_Borne_Diseases/Rocky_Mountain_Spotted_Fever.htm.

38. Florida Department of Health, Tallahassee, "Ehrlichiosis and Anaplasmo-

sis," http://www.doh.state.fl.us/environment/medicine/arboviral/Tick_Borne_Diseases/Human_Ehrlichiosis.htm.

39. Florida Department of Health, Tallahassee, "Southern Tick-Associated Rash Illness," http://www.doh.state.fl.us/Environment/medicine/arboviral/Tick_Borne_Diseases/STARI.html.

40. Florida Department of Health, Tallahassee, "Babesiosis," http://www.doh.state.fl.us/ENVIRONMENT/medicine/arboviral/Tick_Borne_Diseases/Babesiosis.htm.

41. Florida Department of Health, Tallahassee, "Rickettsia parkeri," http://www.doh.state.fl.us/Environment/medicine/arboviral/Tick_Borne_Diseases/Parkeri.html.

42. P. G. Koehler and F. M. Oi, "Ticks," UF/IFAS Extension, February 2003, http://edis.ifas.ufl.edu/IG088.

43. "Lyme Disease," *Health Beat,* Illinois Department of Public Health, http://www.idph.state.il.us/public/hb/hblyme.htm.

44. G. Burke, S. K. Wikel, A. Spielman, S. R. Telford, K. McKay, P. J. Krause, et al., "Hypersensitivity to Ticks and Lyme Disease Risk," *Emerging Infectious Diseases,* 2005, http://www.cdc.gov/ncidod/EID/vol11no01/04–0303.htm.

45. University of Virginia Health System, "Study Describes New Notion in Diagnosing Food Allergies, 'Delayed Anaphylaxis,'" 14 May 2009, http://www.newswise.com/p/articles/view/552423/.

46. "Tick Habitats," *Tick Borne Disease Ecology and Control,* Freehold Township, 2007, http://www.twp.freehold.nj.us/tbde/public/risk_assessment/tick_habitats.asp.

47. Rhode Island Department of Health, "Lyme Disease," 2009, http://www.health.state.ri.us/disease/communicable/lyme/yard.php.

48. Florida Department of Health, Tallahassee, "Tick-borne Disease in Florida," http://www.doh.state.fl.us/Environment/medicine/arboviral/Tick_Borne_Diseases/Tick_Index.htm.

Chapter 9. Assorted Arthropoda

1. John Moffitt, MD, "Allergic Reactions to Insect Stings and Bites," *Southern Medical Journal* 96 (2003): 1073–79.

2. P. Gullan, P. S. Cranston, and Karina Hansen McInnes, *The Insects: An Outline of Entomology* (New York: Wiley-Blackwell, 2004).

3. Mark Deyrup, *Florida's Fabulous Insects* (Hawaiian Gardens, Calif.: World Publications, 2000).

4. Terry Price, "Wheel Bugs, Hazards of the Outdoors," *Forest Pests: Insects, Diseases, and Other Damage Agents,* University of Georgia, April 2006, http://www.forestpests.org/publichealth/wheelbug.html.

5. Elizabeth Radke, MPHH, "Chagas Disease in Florida," *EpiUpdate,* Florida Department of Health, Bureau of Epidemiology, Tallahassee, April 2009.

6. Christopher Paddock et al., "Identification, Cloning, and Recombinant Expression of Procalin, a Major Triatomine Allergen," *Journal of Immunology* 167 (2001): 2694–99.

7. University of Arizona Cooperative Extension, "The Conenose Bug (aka 'The Kissing Bug')," http://ag.arizona.edu/pubs/insects/az1109.pdf.

8. National Pest Management Association, *The NPMA Releases First-Ever Comprehensive Global Bed Bug Study to Determine Extent of Resurgence,* 26 July 2010, http://www.pestworld.org/bedbug.

9. Allison Aubrey, "The Only Good Bedbug Is a Toasted One," National Public Radio, April 2009, http://www.npr.org/templates/story/story.php?storyId=103091338.

10. Joanna Molloy, "BedBug Central Conference Offers Victims Invasive Battlefield Tactics for Dealing with Critters," *New York Daily News,* 22 September 2010.

11. Associated Press, "NYC Looks to Halt Massive Bedbug Infestation," 28 July 2010.

12. P. G. Koehler, R. M. Pereira, M. Pfiester, and Jeff Hertz, *Bed Bugs and Blood-Sucking Conenose,* UF/IFAS Extension, November 2008, http://edis.ifas.ufl.edu/IG083.

13. C. F. Lowe and M. G. Romney, "Bedbugs as Vectors for Drug-Resistant Bacteria," letter, *Emerg Infect Dis.,* June 2011.

14. Mayo Clinic Staff, "Bedbugs," *Mayo Clinic,* December 2007, http://www.mayoclinic.com/health/bedbugs/DS00663.

15. "How Bed Bugs Outsmart Poisons Designed to Control Them," *Newswise Science,* 9 January 2009, http://www.newswise.com/articles/view/547929.

16. John Signore, "Mutant NYC Bed Bugs Impervious to Toxic Attack," *Weblog Gothamist,* January 2009, http://gothamist.com/2009/01/14/mutant_nyc_bed_bugs_impervious_to_p.php.

17. Koehler et al., *Bed Bugs and Blood-Sucking Conenose.*

18. Kimberly Miller, "Turning Up the Heat: Dorm Room Bedbugs Have Enemy in UF Invention," *Palm Beach Post,* 7 July 2009.

19. Aubrey, "The Only Good Bedbug Is a Toasted One."

20. CDC, "Lice," 2008, http://www.cdc.gov/lice/.

21. D. L. Richman and P. G. Koehler, *Fleas: What They Are, What to Do,* UF/IFAS Extension, July 2007. http://edis.ifas.ufl.edu/IG132.

22. Ibid.

23. National Institutes of Health, *Fleas,* Bethesda, Md., 2009, http://www.nlm.nih.gov/medlineplus/ency/article/001329.htm.

24. Richmond and Koehler, *Fleas: What They Are, What to Do.*

25. Moffitt, "Allergic Reactions to Insect Stings and Bites."

26. P. G. Koehler and F. M. Oi, *Biting Flies,* UF/IFAS Extension, April 2003, http://edis.ifas.ufl.edu/IG081.

27. Sean Strother, "Tabanids (Horseflies)," *Dermatology Online Journal,* 1999, http://dermatology.cdlib.org/DOJvol5num2/centerfold/tabanids.html.

28. James E. Cilek, PhD, "The Yellow-Biting Flies of Florida," *EntGuide 1*, Florida A&M University, http://www.pherec.org/EntGuides/EntGuide1.pdf.

29. G. B. Fairchild, H. V. Weems Jr., and T. R. Fasulo, *Yellow Fly, Diachlorus ferrugatus (Fabricius) (Insecta: Diptera: Tabanidae)*, UF/IFAS Extension, April 2004, http://edis.ifas.ufl.edu/IN595.

30. Jason M. Squitier, "Deer Flies, Yellow Flies, and Horse Flies," *Featured Creatures*, UF/IFAS Extension, July 2007, http://entnemdept.ufl.edu/creatures/beneficial/cicada_killers.htm.

31. Fairchild et al., *Yellow Fly*.

32. P. G. Koehler and F. M. Oi, *Control of Biting Flies*, UF/IFAS Extension, April 2003, http://edis.ifas.ufl.edu/IG081; Squitier, "Deer Flies."

33. Dr. Russell F. Mizell, *The Trolling Deer Fly Trap*, North Florida Research and Education Center, December 2009, http://entomology.ifas.ufl.edu/pestalert/deerfly.htm.

34. P. G. Koehler and P. E. Kaufman, *Stable Fly (Dog Fly) Control*, UF/IFAS Extension, July 2006, http://edis.ifas.ufl.edu/IG133.

35. "Allergists Provide Tips to Prevent Bug Bites," *Newswise Medical News*, 15 May 2005, http://www.newswise.com/articles/view/511772.

36. Craig Freudenrich, PhD, "How Mosquitoes Work," *How Stuff Works*, 5 July 2001, http://animals.howstuffworks.com/insects/mosquito.htm.

37. Wayne J. Crans, "Why Mosquitoes Cannot Transmit AIDS," *New Jersey Mosquito Homepage*, Rutgers Cooperative Extension, http://www.rci.rutgers.edu/~insects/aids.htm.

38. Jorge Rey, *The Mosquito*, UF/IFAS Extension, June 2009, http://edis.ifas.ufl.edu/IN652.

39. Florida Medical Entomology Laboratory, University of Florida, *Mosquito Ecology*, http://mosquito.ifas.ufl.edu/Mosquito_Ecology.htm.

40. U.S. Environmental Protection Agency, "DEET," *R.E.D. FACTS*, Cincinnati, National Center for Environmental Publications and Information, April 1998, http://www.epa.gov/oppsrrd1/REDs/factsheets/0002fact.pdf.

41. Ibid.

42. C. D. Morris, PhD, and J. F. Day, PhD, *Avoiding and Repelling Mosquitoes*, Collier Mosquito Control District, March 1993, http://www.collier-mosquito.org/pdfs/avoiding_mosquitoes.pdf.

43. Roxanne C. Rutledge and Jonathan F. Day, *Biting Midges of Coastal Florida*, UF/IFAS Extension, May 2008, http://edis.ifas.ufl.edu/MG102.

44. Koehler and Oi, *Control of Biting Flies*.

45. P. D. Armitage, L. C. Pinder, and P. S. Cranston, *Chironomidae: The Biology and Ecology of Non-Biting Midges* (New York: Springer, 1995).

46. Rutledge and Day, *Biting Midges of Coastal Florida*.

47. Roxanne C. Rutledge-Connelly, "Biting Midges, No-See-Ums," *Featured Creatures*, UF/IFAS Extension, May 2005, http://entomology.ifas.ufl.edu/creatures/aquatic/biting_midges.htm.

48. Ibid.

49. Phadia, *Green nimitti,* http://www.phadia.com/en/Allergen-information/ImmunoCAP-Allergens/Insects/Allergens/Green-nimitti.

50. Koehler and Oi, *Control of Biting Flies.*

51. Charles Apperson, Michael Waldvogel, and Stephen Bambara, "Biology and Control of Non-Biting Aquatic Midges," *Residential Structural and Community Pests,* North Carolina Cooperative Extension, July 2006, http://www.ces.ncsu.edu/depts/ent/notes/Urban/midges.htm.

52. Armitage et al., *Chironomidae.*

53. Phadia, *Green nimitti.*

54. Apperson et al., "Biology and Control of Non-Biting Aquatic Midges."

55. Phadia, *Green nimitti.*

56. Armitage et al., *Chironomidae.*

57. Apperson et al., "Biology and Control of Non-Biting Aquatic Midges."

58. Jerome Goddard, *Physician's Guide to Arthropods of Medical Importance.* (CRC, 2007).

59. Ross Arnett Jr., "False Blister Beetles," *Featured Creatures,* UF/IFAS Extension, August 2008, http://www.entnemdept.ufl.edu/creatures/urban/medical/false_blister_beetles.htm.

60. John Capinera, "Striped Blister Beetle," *Featured Creatures,* UF/IFAS Extension, January 2003, http://entomology.ifas.ufl.edu/creatures/veg/potato/striped_blister_beetle.htm.

61. Arnett, "False Blister Beetles."

62. Capinera, "Striped Blister Beetle."

63. Arnett, "False Blister Beetles."

64. Ibid.

65. Capinera, "Striped Blister Beetle."

66. Robert Norris, MD, "Caterpillar Envenomation," *eMedicine,* November 2008, http://emedicine.medscape.com/article/772949-overview.

67. D. E. Short, H. Habeck, and J. L. Castner, "Stinging and Venomous Caterpillars," UF/IFAS Extension, June 2005, http://edis.ifas.ufl.edu/IN014.

68. Poison Control Center, University of Miami School of Medicine, *Stinging Caterpillars,* June 2005, http://www.med.miami.edu/poisoncontrol/x54.xml.

69. Eileen Buss and Albert E. Mayfield, *Caterpillars That Defoliate Trees and Shrubs,* UF/IFAS Extension, June 2005, http://edis.ifas.ufl.edu/IN628.

Part III. Allergies in the Garden of Eden

1. William Bartram, *Travels through North and South Carolina, Georgia, East and West Florida, the Cherokee Country, the Extensive Territories of the Muscogulges or Creek Confederacy, and the Country of the Chactaws. Containing an Account of the Soil and Natural Productions of Those Regions; Together with Observations on the Manners of the Indians* (Philadelphia: James and Johnson, 1791).

2. William Bartram, *Travels of William Bartram* (New York: Cosimo, 2007), 15.

3. Ibid., 186.

Chapter 10. Look but Don't Touch

1. Christina Marino, "Phytodermatitis: Reactions in the Skin Caused by Plants," *Safety & Health Assessment & Research for Prevention Report* 63 (2001).

2. Kyle Moppert, *Nasties, Beasties, and Things That'll 'Git Cha,'* Center for Environmental Health Services Office of Public Health, Louisiana Department of Health, 2008, http://www.docstoc.com/docs/2495069/Nasties-and-beasties-and-things1.

3. University of Florida School of Forest Resources and Conservation, "Pricklypear (Opuntia humifusa)," *Florida Forest Plants*, http://www.sfrc.ufl.edu/4h/Prickly_pear/pricpear.htm.

4. Dan Culbert, *Prickley Pear for Pain and Pleasure*, UF/IFAS Okeechobee County Extension Service, 2006, http://okeechobee.ifas.ufl.edu/News%20columns/Prickley.Pear.htm.

5. Herbert P. Goodheart and Arthur C. Huntley, "Cactus Dermatitis," *Dermatology Online Journal*, 2001, http://dermatology.cdlib.org/DOJvol7num2/unknown/cholla/cholla2.html.

6. J. A. Ferrell and B. A. Sellers, *Blackberry and Dewberry: Biology and Control*, University of Florida IFAS Extension, Florida Cooperative Extension Service, Institute of Food and Agricultural Sciences, University of Florida (hereafter UF/IFAS Extension), November 2010, http://edis.ifas.ufl.edu/AG238.

7. Lewis Cozen and Maxwell Fonda, "Palm Thorn Injuries: Difficulty in Diagnosis of Late Sequelae," *California Medicine* 79 (1953): 40, 41.

8. Pieter van der Valk, *The Irritant Contact Dermatitis Syndrome (Dermatology: Clinical & Basic Science)*, Informa HealthCare, 1995.

9. Modi et al., "Irritant Contact Dermatitis from Plants."

10. Glen H. Crawford, MD, "Botanical Dermatology," *eMedicine*, WebMD, 2007, http://emedicine.medscape.com/article/1090097-overview.

11. New Zealand Dermatological Society, "Urticaria," *Dermnet NZ*, 2009, http://dermnetnz.org/reactions/urticaria.html.

12. Smita Amin, Howard I. Maibach, and Arto Lahti, *Contact Urticaria Syndrome (Dermatology: Clinical & Basic Science)*, Informa HealthCare, 1997.

13. Wendy B. Zomlefer, "Stinging Nettles of Florida: Urtica," UF/IFAS Extension, 2008, http://edis.ifas.ufl.edu/HB002.

14. University of Maryland Medical Center, "Stinging Nettle," *Complementary Medicine*, 2009, http://www.umm.edu/altmed/articles/stinging-nettle-000275.htm.

15. "How to Cope with a Warmer World," *Consumer Reports*, June 2009.

16. A. S. Stibich, M. Yagan, V. Sharma, B. Herndon, and C. A. Montgomery,

"Cost-Effective Post-Exposure Prevention of Poison Ivy Dermatitis," *International Journal of Dermatology Treatment* 39 (7): 515–18.

17. Aetna Intellihealth, "Poison Ivy: Prevention and Treatment," *Allergy*, December 2009, http://www.intelihealth.com/IH/ihtIH/WSIHW000/7945/8214/7770.html?d=dmtJHE.

18. Internet Dermatology Society, "Allergic Contact Dermatitis," *Electronic Textbook of Dermatology*, 2000, http://telemedicine.org/botanica/bot6.htm.

19. Klilah Hershko, Ido Weinberg, and Arieh Ingber, "Exploring the Mango–Poison Ivy Connection: The Riddle of Discriminative Plant Dermatitis," *Contact Dermatitis* 52 (2005): 3–5.

20. Internet Dermatology Society, "Allergic Contact Dermatitis."

21. Steve Christman, "Schinus terebinthifolius," *Floridata*, 2004, http://www.floridata.com/ref/S/schi_ter.cfm.

22. University of Florida 4H Forest Ecology, "Poisonwood (*Metopium toxiferum*)," *Florida Forest Trees*, http://www.sfrc.ufl.edu/4h/poisonwood/poisonwo.htm.

23. Steven D. Ehrlich, "Dandelion," *Complementary Medicine*, University of Maryland Medical Center, 5 December 2008, http://www.umm.edu/altmed/articles/dandelion-000236.htm.

24. Internet Dermatology Society, "Allergic Contact Dermatitis."

25. Ibid.

26. William P. Baugh, "Phytophotodermatitis," *eMedicine*, *WebMD*, 2007, http://emedicine.medscape.com/article/1119566-overview.

27. New Zealand Dermatological Society, "PUVA (Photochemotherapy)," *DermNet NZ*, 2009, http://dermnetnz.org/procedures/puva.html.

Chapter 11. Stop to Smell the Roses but Take Shallow Breaths

1. Neil Osterweil, "AAAAI: Seasonal Allergy Patients Also Bugged by Non-Allergic Irritants," *MedPage Today*, 1 March 2007, http://www.medpagetoday.com/MeetingCoverage/AAAAI/5146.

2. Thomas Leo Ogren, "Allergy-Free in the Rose Garden," *Garden Forever*, http://www.gardenforever.com/pages/artallergy.htm.

3. V. Mahillon, S. Saussez, and O. Michel, "High Incidence of Sensitization to Ornamental Plants in Allergic Rhinitis," *Allergy* 61, no. 9 (September 2006): 1138–40.

4. Ibid.

5. P. Gaig, B. Bartolome, E. Enrique, P. Garcia-Ortega, and R. Palacios, "Hypersensitivity to *Ficus benjamina*," *Spanish Society of Allergy and Clinical Immunology* 14, no. 4 (1999): 212–17.

6. J. M. De Greefa, F. Lieutier-Colasb, J. C. Bessotb, A. Vérotb, A. M. Gallerandc, G. Paulib, and F. de Blayb, "Urticaria and Rhinitis to Shrubs of *Ficus benjamina* and

Breadfruit in a Banana-Allergic Road Worker: Evidence for a Cross-Sensitization between Moracea, Banana, and Latex," *International Archives of Allergy and Immunology* 125 (2001): 182–84.

7. Thomas Leo Ogren, "Allergy-free Wedding Flowers," *Garden Forever,* http://www.gardenforever.com/pages/artwedding.htm.

8. Ibid.

9. Mayo Clinic, "Non-Allergic Rhinitis," 7 August 2008, http://www.mayoclinic.com/health/nonallergic-rhinitis/DS00809.

10. Rondón et al. "Evolution of Non-Allergic Rhinitis Supports Conversion to Allergic Rhinitis," *JACI Highlights* 123, no. 5 (May 2009), http://www.aaaai.org/patients/jaci/content.asp?contentid=8782.

11. Osterweil, "AAAAI."

12. Mayo Clinic, "Non-Allergic Rhinitis."

Chapter 12. Why Does My Tongue Itch?

1. Theresa Willingham, *Food Allergy Field Guide: A Lifestyle Manual for Families* (Littleton, Col.: Savory Palate, 2nd ed., 2006)

2. Takeshi Yagami, "Allergies to Cross-Reactive Plant Proteins: Latex-Fruit Syndrome Is Comparable with Pollen-Food Allergy Syndrome," *International Archives of Allergy and Immunology* 128, no. 4 (2002): 271–79.

3. Food Allergy and Anaphylaxis Network, "What Is a Food Allergy?" 2009, http://www.foodallergy.org/questions.html.

4. Royal Brompton and Harefield NHS Trust, "The Diagnosis of Oral Allergy Syndrome through the Use of a Structured Questionnaire," 2009, Clinical Trials.gov.

5. Salynn Boyles, "Treating Allergies with Allergic Food," *WebMD*, 2006, http://www.webmd.com/allergies/news/20061128/food-allergies-possibly-treated-with-allergic-food.

6. Yagami, "Allergies to Cross-Reactive Plant Proteins."

7. Jonathan H. Crane, Carlos F. Balerdi, and Ian Maguire, "Avocado Growing in the Florida Home Landscape," *University of Florida IFAS Extension,* Florida Cooperative Extension Service, Institute of Food and Agricultural Sciences, University of Florida (hereafter UF/IFAS Extension), August 2007, http://edis.ifas.ufl.edu/MG213; Dr. Harris Steinman, "Avocado," Phadia, http://www.phadia.com/en-US/Allergens/ImmunoCAP-Allergens/Food-of-Plant-Origin/Vegetables/Avocado-/.

8. California Avocados, "Avocado Nutrition Structure/Function Statements," 2009, http://www.avocado.org/healthy-living/nutrition.

9. Jonathan H. Crane, Carlos F. Balerdi, and Ian Maguire, "Banana Growing in the Florida Home Landscape," UF/IFAS Extension, October 2008,http://edis.ifas.ufl.edu/MG040.

10. Dr. Harris Steinman, "Banana," Phadia, 2008, http://www.phadia.com/en-US/Allergens/ImmunoCAP-Allergens/Food-of-Plant-Origin/Fruits/Banana/.

11. Dr. Harris Steinman, "Cashew Nut." Phadia, 2008, http://www.phadia.com/en-US/Allergens/ImmunoCAP-Allergens/Food-of-Plant-Origin/Seeds-Nuts/Cashew-nut-/.

12. Edward F. Gilman and Dennis G. Watson, "Litchi chinensis: Lychee," UF/IFAS Extension, March 2007, http://edis.ifas.ufl.edu/ST364.

13. Dr. Harris Steinman, "Litchi," Phadia, 2008, http://www.phadia.com/en-US/Allergens/ImmunoCAP-Allergens/Food-of-Plant-Origin/Fruits/Litchi/.

14. Ogren, *Allergy-Free Gardening*.

15. Jonathan H. Crane, Carlos F. Balerdi, and Ian Maguire. "Mango Growing in the Florida Home Landscape." UF/IFAS Extension, November 2006, http://edis.ifas.ufl.edu/MG216.

16. Dr. Harris Steinman, "Mango," Phadia, 2008, http://www.phadia.com/en-US/Allergens/ImmunoCAP-Allergens/Food-of-Plant-Origin/Fruits/Mango/.

17. Jonathan Crane, "Papaya Growing in the Florida Home Landscape," UF/IFAS Extension, October 2008, http://edis.ifas.ufl.edu/MG054.

18. Ogren, *Allergy-Free Gardening* (papaya plants are pollen-free); Dr. Harris Steinman, "Papaya," Phadia, 2008, http://www.phadia.com/en-US/Allergens/ImmunoCAP-Allergens/Food-of-Plant-Origin/Fruits/Papaya/.

19. Ginger M. Allen, Michael D. Bond, and Martin B. Main, "50 Common Native Plants Important in Florida," UF/IFAS Extension, August 2009, http://edis.ifas.ufl.edu/UW152.

20. Torsten Ulmer and John M. MacDougal, *Passiflora: Passionflowers of the World* (Portland, Ore.: Timber Press, 2004).

21. Dr. Harris Steinman, "Passion Fruit," Phadia, 2000, http://www.phadia.com/en-US/Allergens/ImmunoCAP-Allergens/Food-of-Plant-Origin/Fruits/Passion-fruit/.

22. Dr. Harris Steinman, "Pineapple," Phadia, 2008, http://www.phadia.com/en-US/Allergens/ImmunoCAP-Allergens/Food-of-Plant-Origin/Fruits/Pineapple/.

23. Clifford W. Bassett, MD, and Ilana Bragin, MD, "Ragweed and Oral Allergy Syndrome," *American Academy of Allergy Asthma & Immunology*, 2009, http://www.aaaai.org/patients/advocate/2007/fall/ragweed.asp.

24. Calgary Allergy Network, "Botanical Food Family List," http://www.calgaryallergy.ca/Articles/English/botanical.htm.

25. Florida Department of Citrus, "Citrus Facts," 2008, http://www.floridajuice.com/juice.php.

26. Dr. Harris Steinman, "Grapefruit," Phadia, 2008, http://www.phadia.com/en-US/Allergens/ImmunoCAP-Allergens/Food-of-Plant-Origin/Fruits/Grape-fruit/.

27. Dr. Harris Steinman, "Orange," Phadia, 2008, http://www.phadia.com/en-US/Allergens/ImmunoCAP-Allergens/Food-of-Plant-Origin/Fruits/Orange/

28. Ibid.

29. Jonathan H. Crane, "Carambola Growing in the Florida Home Landscape," UF/IFAS Extension, May 2007, http://edis.ifas.ufl.edu/MG269.

30. Dr. Harris Steinman, "Carambola," Phadia, 2008, http://www.phadia.com/en-US/Allergens/ImmunoCAP-Allergens/Food-of-Plant-Origin/Fruits/Carambola/.

31. Miguel Moyses Neto, MD, "Star Fruit Intoxication in Uraemic Patients," *Cin*, 2003, http://www.uninet.edu/cin2003/conf/mmoyses/mmoyses.html.

32. Timothy K. Broschat and Jonathan H. Crane, "The Coconut Palm in Florida," UF/IFAS Extension, December 2008, http://edis.ifas.ufl.edu/MG043.

33. Dr. Harris Steinman, "Coconut," Phadia, 2008, http://www.phadia.com/en-US/Allergens/ImmunoCAP-Allergens/Food-of-Plant-Origin/Seeds-Nuts/Coconut-/.

34. Jonathan H. Crane and Carlos F. Balerdi, "Guava Growing in the Florida Home Landscape," UF/IFAS Extension, 2005, http://edis.ifas.ufl.edu/MG045.

35. Dr. Harris Steinman, "Guava," Phadia, 2008, http://www.phadia.com/en-US/Allergens/ImmunoCAP-Allergens/Food-of-Plant-Origin/Fruits/Guava/.

36. Florida Strawberry Growers Association, "History," 2009, http://www.flastrawberry.com/history.aspx.

37. Dr. Harris Steinman, "Strawberry," Phadia, 2008, http://www.phadia.com/en-US/Allergens/ImmunoCAP-Allergens/Food-of-Plant-Origin/Fruits/Strawberry/.

Part IV. The Life Aquatic

1. David McRee, http://www.beachhunter.net/download/florida-beach-safety-v-2011-3.pdf.

2. "Florida's State Park Attendance Reaches New Heights," Department of Environmental Protection, 2009, http://www.dep.state.fl.us/secretary/news/2009/07/0722_01.htm.

3. Earthdive.com, "Florida Straits—Most Diverse Marine Life in Atlantic," August 2003, http://www.earthdive.com/site/news/newsdetail.asp?id=228.

4. Smithsonian Marine Station at Fort Pierce, "Indian River Lagoon Species Index," August 2003, http://www.sms.si.edu/irlspec/index.htm.

5. Florida Department of Health, "Epidemiology of Unintentional Drownings in Florida, 2001–2005," 2006, http://www.doh.state.fl.us/Injury/DrownPrevent.html.

6. Florida Fish and Wildlife Conservation Commission, "Boating Accident Statistics," 2008, http://myfwc.com/SAFETY/Safety_Boat_Safety_AccidentStats.htm.

Chapter 13. The Sting of Cnidaria

1. Allen Collins, "Jellyfish, Corals, and Other Stingers," *Introduction to Cnidaria,* University of California Museum of Paleontology, April 2001, http://www.ucmp. berkeley.edu/cnidaria/cnidaria.html.

2. Paul S. Auerbach, "Stinging Truths, Part 1: A Guide to Injuries Caused by Invertebrates," *Dive Training Magazine,* http://www.dtmag.com/Stories/Dive%20 Medicine/02–96-dive_medicine.htm.

3. Robert Barish, "Marine Bites and Stings," *Merck Manuals Online Medical Library,* February 2009, http://www.merck.com/mmpe/sec21/ch325/ch325f.html.

4. David R. Boulware, "A Randomized, Controlled Field Trial for the Prevention of Jellyfish Stings with a Topical Sting Inhibitor," *Journal of Travel Medicine* 13, no. 3 (2007): 166–71.

5. Patricia J. Garcia, Roland M. H. Schein, and Joseph W. Burnett, "Fulminant Hepatic Failure from a Sea Anemone Sting Trial for the Prevention of Jellyfish Stings with a Topical Sting Inhibitor," *Annals of Internal Medicine* 120, no. 8 (1994): 665–66.

6. "Jellyfish Sting Hundreds at Central Florida Beach," WFTV, August 2007, http://www.wftv.com/news/13822837/detail.html.

7. Coalition on the Public Understanding of Science, "Meet the Bonaire Banded Box Jellyfish," *Year of Science 2009,* http://www.yearofscience2009.org/themes_ ocean_water/general/meet-bbbj.html.

8. J. Grady and J. Burnett, "Irukandji-like Syndrome in South Florida Divers," *Annals of Emergency Medicine* 42, no. 6 (2003): 763–66.

9. Patrick G. Daubert, M.D., "Cnidaria Envenomation," *eMedicine,* WebMD, August 2008, http://emedicine.medscape.com/article/769538-overview.

10. Richard A. Clinchy III, *Dive-First Responder* (St. Louis: Mosby Lifeline, 1996).

11. Arlen Stauffer, and Paul S. Auerbach, "Marine Envenomations: Florida Related Injuries and Illnesses," *EMpulse* 8.3.2 (2003): 11–14, http://www.buysafesea. com/EMpulse1.pdf.

12. Clinchy, *Dive-First Responder.*

13. Daubert, "Cnidaria Envenomation."

14. Edwin S. Iversen and Renate H. Skinner, *Dangerous Sea Life of the West Atlantic, Caribbean, and Gulf of Mexico* (Sarasota, Fla.: Pineapple Press, 2006).

15. Kate Spinner, "Jellyfish Inundate Southwest Florida Bays; Drought May Be to Blame," *Herald-Tribune,* 4 December 2007.

16. "Upside-down Jellyfish," Marine Invertebrates of Bermuda, Bermuda Institute of Ocean Sciences, http://www.thecephalopodpage.org/MarineInvertebrate-Zoology/Cassiopeaxamachana.html.

17. "Cannonball Jellyfish," *Florida Seafood.com,* 2004, http://www.fl-seafood. com/species/jellyfish.htm.

18. Iversen and Skinner, *Dangerous Sea Life.*

19. "Jellyfish!" *University of Florida Institute of Food and Agricultural Sciences AquaNotes,* 2007.

20. Iversen and Skinner, *Dangerous Sea Life.*

21. Clarence William Brown Jr., M.D., "Seabather's Eruption," *eMedicine,* WebMD, May 2008, http://emedicine.medscape.com/article/1088160-overview.

22. Marine Species Identification Portal, "Fire Coral," *ETI BioInformatics,* http://species-identification.org/search.php?search_for=fire+coral&x=0&y=0.

23. Elizabeth K. Gocek, "Milleporina: The Fire Coral; Development and Importance of Fire Coral," *Tropical Ecosystems,* Miami University, May 2002, http://jrscience.wcp.muohio.edu/FieldCourses00/PapersMarineEcologyArticles/Milleporina.TheFireCoralD.html.

24. Marine Species Identification Portal, "Fire Coral."

25. Clinchy, *Dive-First Responder.*

26. Mindy B. Kurlansky, "*Physalia physalis,*" *Animal Diversity Web,* 2002, http://animaldiversity.ummz.umich.edu/site/accounts/information/Physalia_physalis.html.

27. Miranda Hoover, "Portuguese Man-of-War (*Physalia physalis*)," *Marine Invertebrates of Bermuda,* Bermuda Institute of Ocean Sciences, http://www.thecephalopodpage.org/MarineInvertebrateZoology/Physaliaphysalis.html.

28. Daubert, "Cnidaria Envenomation."

29. Stauffer and Auerbach, Marine Envenomations."

30. Auerbach, "Stinging Truths."

31. Daubert, "Cnidaria Envenomation."

32. Brown, "Seabather's Eruption."

33. Clinchy, *Dive-First Responder.*

34. Paul Auerbach, M.D., "Medicine for the Outdoors," *Healthline,* 29 April 2009, http://www.healthline.com/blogs/outdoor_health/labels/marine%20envenomation.html.

35. Stauffer and Auerbach, "Marine Envenomations."

Chapter 14. Doing the Stingray Shuffle

1. Zoltan Trizna, "Cutaneous Manifestations Following Exposures to Marine Life," *eMedicine,* WebMD, February 2009, http://emedicine.medscape.com/article/1089144-overview.

2. Wheeler C. Ward and William Leo Smith, "Venom Evolution Widespread in Fishes: A Phylogenetic Road Map for the Bioprospecting of Piscine Venoms," *Journal of Heredity* 97, no. 3 (2006): 206–17.

3. Vidal Haddad Jr., Pedro Pereira Oliveira Pardal, João Luiz Costa Cardoso, and Itamar Alves Marteis, "The Venomous Toadfish Thalassophryne nattereri," *Revista do Instituto de Medicina Tropical de São Paulo* 45, no. 4 (July/August 2003): 221–23.

4. Edwin S. Iversen and Renate H. Skinner, *Dangerous Sea Life of the West Atlantic, Caribbean, and Gulf of Mexico* (Sarasota, Fla.: Pineapple Press, 2006).

5. Casey Patton, "Southern Stargazer," *Ichthyology,* Florida Museum of Natural History, http://www.flmnh.ufl.edu/fish/gallery/descript/stargazersouth/stargazer-south.htm.

6. "Venomous Marine Animals," *Texas Sea Grant,* Texas A&M University, http://texas-sea-grant.tamu.edu/online%20publications/Venomous%20Poster.pdf.

7. Jacqui Goddard, "Lionfish Devastate Florida's Native Shoals," *Times Online,* 20 October 2008.

8. Florida Fish and Wildlife Conservation Commission, Fish and Wildlife Research Institute (FWRI), "First-Known Lionfish Caught in Florida's Gulf Coast Waters," 2006, http://research.myfwc.com/features/view_article.asp?id=27520.

9. Scott A. Gallagher, "Lionfish and Stonefish," *eMedicine,* WebMD, 2 December 2008, http://emedicine.medscape.com/article/770764-overview.

10. "Venomous Marine Animals."

11. Florida Fish and Wildlife Conservation Commission, "Fish ID: Freshwater," http://myfwc.com/WILDLIFEHABITATS/Freshwater_Fish_ID.htm.

12. Suzanne Shepherd, Stephen H. Thomas, and C. Keith Stone, "Catfish Envenomation," *Journal of Wilderness Medicine* 5, no. 1 (1994): 67–70.

13. Nadeem Ajmal, Lillian B. Nanney, and Sean F. Wolfort, "Catfish Spine Envenomation: A Case of Delayed Presentation," *Wilderness and Environmental Medicine* 14, no. 2 (2003): 101–105.

14. "Venomous Marine Animals."

15. Ibid.

16. "International Shark Attack File," *Ichthyology,* Florida Museum of Natural History, http://www.flmnh.ufl.edu/fish/sharks/isaf/graphs.htm#flshark.

17. "Spiny Dogfish (*Squalus acanthias*)," *ARKive,* 2008, http://www.arkive.org/spiny-dogfish/squalus-acanthias/info.html.

18. Al Kline, D.P.M., "Stingray Envenomation of the Foot: A Case Report," *Foot and Ankle Journal* 6, no. 4 (2008).

19. Mote Marine Laboratory, "About Stingrays," http://www.mote.org/index.php?src=gendocs&ref=Stingrays&category=Shark%20Research.

20. Arlen R. Stauffer, M.D., M.B.A., and Paul S. Auerbach, M.D., M.S., " Marine Envenomations: Florida Related Injuries and Illnesses," *EMpulse* 8.3.2 (2003): 11–14, http://www.buysafesea.com/EMpulse1.pdf.

21. Kline, "Stingray Envenomation of the Foot."

22. Steve Grenard, "Stingray Injuries, Envenomation, and Medical Management," http://www.potamotrygon.de/fremdes/stingray%20article.htm.

23. David DuBois, M.D., "Stingray Injury," *eMedicine,* WebMD, 2005, http://www.emedicinehealth.com/stingray_injury/article_em.htm.

24. BioMedia Associates, "Branches on the Tree of Life: Echinoderms," http://ebiomedia.com/prod/BOechinoderms.html.

25. Barbara Drobina, D.O., "Dive Medicine: Sea Urchin Puncture Wound," *eMedicine,* http://www.emedicinehealth.com/wilderness_sea_urchin_puncture/article_em.htm.

26. Richard V. Aghababian, ed., *Essentials of Emergency Medicine* (Sudbury, Mass.: Jones and Bartlett, 2006.

27. Scott A. Gallagher, M.D., F.A.C.E.P., "Echinoderm Envenomation," *eMedicine,* http://emedicine.medscape.com/article/770053-overview.

28. Scott H. Plantz, M.D., F.A.A.E.M., "Sea Cucumber Irritation," *eMedicine,* http://www.emedicinehealth.com/wilderness_sea_cucumber_irritation/article_em.htm.

29. Gallagher, "Echinoderm Envenomation."

30. Marine Species Identification Portal, "Greater Soapfish (*Rypticus saponaceus*)," *Interactive Guide to Caribbean Diving,* http://species-identification.org/species.php?species_group=caribbean_diving_guide&id=194.

31. James R. Warpinski, M.D., Jeffrey Folgert, B.S., Martin Voss, M.D., and Robert K. Bush, M.D., "Fish Surface Mucin Hypersensitivity," *Journal of Wilderness Medicine* 4, no. 3 (1993): 261–69.

32. L. H. Sweat, "Fire Sponge," Smithsonian Marine Station at Ft. Pierce, http://www.sms.si.edu/IRLSpec/Tedani_ignis.htm.

33. Lewis R. Goldfrank, Neal Flomenbaum, Neal Lewin, Mary Ann Howland, Robert Hoffman, and Lewis Nelson, *Goldfrank's Toxicologic Emergencies,* 7th ed. (New York: McGraw-Hill Professional, 2002).

34. William Burke, "Cutaneous Reactions to Marine Sponges and Bryozoans," *Dermatologic Therapy* 15, no. 1 (2002): 26–29.

35. Richard A. Clinchy, *Dive-First Responder* (St. Louis: Mosby Lifeline, 1996).

Chapter 15. Sun and Sea: A Day at the Beach

1. Florida Fish and Wildlife Conservation Commission (FWCC), "Fast Facts," 2009, http://myfwc.com/About/About_FastFacts.htm.

2. G. M. Abbott, J. H. Landsberg, A. R. Reich, K. A. Steidinger, S. Ketchen, and C. Blackmore, *Resource Guide for Public Health Response to Harmful Algal Blooms in Florida,* Florida Fish and Wildlife Conservation Commission, Fish and Wildlife Research Institute Technical Report TR-14, 2009, http://research.myfwc.com/publications/publication_info.asp?id=58596.

3. Robert J. MacNeal, "Photosensitivity Reactions," *Merck Manual of Medical Information,* 2nd ed., August 2007, http://www.merck.com/mmhe/print/sec18/ch214/ch214c.html.

4. Mayo Clinic staff, "Sun Allergy," 29 April 2010, http://www.mayoclinic.com/health/sun-allergy/DS01178/DSECTION=prevention.

5. Ibid.

6. Smithsonian Museum of Natural History, "Algae Research," 2010, http://botany.si.edu/projects/algae/introduction.htm.

7. Centers for Disease Control (CDC), "Harmful Algal Blooms: Facts about Cyanobacteria and Cyanobacterial Harmful Algal Blooms," 2004, http://www.cdc.gov/hab/cyanobacteria/facts.htm.

8. "Blue-Green Algae," *Wellness Guide to Dietary Supplements,* University of California at Berkley, 2010, http://www.wellnessletter.com/html/ds/dsBlueGreen-Algae.php.

9. Abbott et al., *Resource Guide.*

10. CDC, "Harmful Algal Blooms."

11. FWCC, "Fast Facts."

12. Abbott et al., *Resource Guide.*

13. Ibid.

14. Dana Bigham, "Toxic Algae: Should Floridians Be Worried?" *Florida Lakewatch* 42 (2008): 1–3.

15. Craig Pitman, "Red Tide Study Shows Toxins, Potential Benefits," *St. Petersburg Times,* 25 March 2011.

16. Sharon Watkins, Andrew Reich, Lora E. Fleming, and Roberta Hammond, "Neurotoxic Shellfish Poisoning," *Marine Drugs* 6 (2008): 431–55.

17. Bigham, "Toxic Algae."

18. J. M. Burkholder and H. B. Glasgow Jr., *"Pfiesteria/Pseudopfiesteria* Fact Sheet," Florida Fish and Wildlife Conservation Commission, Fish and Wildlife Research Institute.

19. CDC, "Harmful Algal Blooms."

20. Jennifer Jurado and Gary Hitchcock, "The Plume and the Bloom," *Florida Baywatch Report* (2001), http://nsgl.gso.uri.edu/flsgp/flsgpg01006.pdf.

21. Florida Fish and Wildlife Conservation Commission, Fish and Wildlife Research Institute (FWRI), "Florida East Coast Diatom Bloom," 15 May 2009, http://myfwc.com/research/redtide/events/other/e-fl-coast-diatom-bloom/.

22. CDC, "What Are Recreational Water Illnesses (RWIs)?" 2007, http://www.cdc.gov/healthywater/swimming/rwi/rwi-what.html.

23. Debra Goldschmidt, "1,800 Infected; Water Park Blamed," *CNN* 20 August 2005, http://articles.cnn.com/2005-08-19/us/water.illness_1_health-department-diarrheal-disease-health-care-workers?_s=PM:US.

24. CDC, "Hot Tub Rash," Pseudomonas Dermatitis/Folliculitis," 2010, http://www.cdc.gov/healthywater/swimming/rwi/illnesses/hot-tub-rash.html.

25. Charles Toner, M.D., *"Pseudomonas* Folliculitis," *MedScape,* WebMD, June 2009, http://emedicine.medscape.com/article/1053170-overview.

26. Barry J. Zacherle, M.D., and Diane S. Silver, M.D., "Hot Tub Folliculitis: A Clinical Syndrome," *Western Journal of Medicine* 137, no. 3 (1982): 191–94.

27. CDC, "Parasites—Naegleria," 2 November 2010, http://www.cdc.gov/parasites/naegleria/.

28. CDC, "Parasites—Cercarial Dermatitis (also known as Swimmer's Itch)," 2 November 2010, http://www.cdc.gov/parasites/swimmersitch/.

Chapter 16. Neptune's Revenge: Seafood Allergies

1. Florida Department of Agriculture and Consumer Services, "Florida Seafood Varieties," 2004, http://www.fl-seafood.com/species/index.htm.

2. Food Allergy & Anaphylaxis Network (FAAN), Mount Sinai Medical Center, "Seafood Allergies Often Begin Later in Life," 9 July 2004, http://www.medicalnewstoday.com/articles/10491.php.

3. National Oceanographic and Atmospheric Administration, "Americans Ate More Seafood in 2002," 2003, http://www.publicaffairs.noaa.gov/releases2003/sep03/noaa03105.html.

4. Canadian Food Inspection Agency, "Seafood (Fish, Crustaceans, and Shellfish)—One of the Nine Most Common Food Allergens," 2009, http://www.inspection.gc.ca/english/fssa/labeti/allerg/fispoie.shtml.

5. "Food Allergens: Fish," Phadia, http://www.phadia.com/en-US/Allergens/Common-Allergens-in-Brief/Food-Allergens/#Fish/.

6. Foti Caterina, Eustacio Nettis, Nicoletta Cassano, Iris Demundo, and Gina Vena, "Acute Allergic Reactions to *Anisakis simplex* after Ingestion of Anchovies," *Acta Dermato-Venereologica* 82 (2002): 12–123.

7. Auckland Allergy Clinic, "Seafood Allergy," February 2003, http://www.allergyclinic.co.nz/guides/51.html.

8. Ibid.

9. "Food Allergens: Fish," Phadia.

10. Cheryl Levin and Erin Warshaw, "Protein Contact Dermatitis," *eMedicine,* 25 June 2009, http://emedicine.medscape.com/article/1604561-overview; Auckland Allergy Clinic, "Seafood Allergy."

11. G. Reese, R. Ayuso, and S. B. Lehrer, "Tropomyosin: An Invertebrate Pan-Allergen," *International Archives of Allergy and Immunology* 119, no. 4 (August 1999): 247–58.

12. Auckland Allergy Clinic, "Seafood Allergy."

13. Peter N. Huynh, "Exercise-Induced Anaphylaxis," *eMedicine,* 16 July 2010, http://emedicine.medscape.com/article/886641-overview.

14. Auckland Allergy Group, "Seafood Allergy."

15. Andreas L. Lopata and Samuel B. Lehrer, "New Insights into Seafood Allergy," *Current Opinion in Allergy and Clinical Immunology* 9, no. 3 (30 July 2009): 270–77.

16. Auckland Allergy Clinic, "Seafood Allergy."

17. S. A. Reid and Christian Boone, "Wife: Man Who Died Didn't Order Crab Dish," *Atlanta Journal Constitution,* 7 July 2008.

18. "Avoiding Hidden Safety Risks with Fatty Fish and Omega-3 Fish Oil Supplements," *Pharmacist's Letter,* Therapeutic Research Center, 13 August 2007, http://bit.ly/et4xab.

19. Australasian Society of Clinical Immunology and Allergy, "Allergic and Toxic Reactions to Seafood," 1 June 2010, http://www.allergy.org.au/aer/infobulletins/seafood_allergy.htm.

20. Anahad O'Connor, "The Claim: If You Have a Seafood Allergy, Avoid CT Scans," *New York Times,* 18 January 2010, http://www.nytimes.com/2010/01/19/health/19real.html.

21. E. Schabelman and M. Witting, "The Relationship of Radiocontrast, Iodine, and Seafood," National Center for Biotechnology Information, 2010, http://www.ncbi.nlm.nih.gov/pubmed/20045605.

22. Food Allergy and Anaphylaxis Network, "Shellfish," http://www.foodallergy.org/page/shellfish1.

23. Auckland Allergy Clinic, "Seafood Allergy."

24. Florida Poison Information Center, University of Miami Leonard M. Miller School of Medicine, "Ciguatera," http://miamipoisoncenter.org/x62.xml.

25. CDC, "Marine Toxins, General Information; CDC Bacterial, Mycotic Diseases," 12 October 2005, http://www.cdc.gov/ncidod/dbmd/diseaseinfo/marinetoxins_g.htm.

26. Florida Poison Information Center, University of Miami Leonard M. Miller School of Medicine, "Puffer Fish Poisoning," http://miamipoisoncenter.org/x64.xml.

Directory of Useful Online Resources

Part I. Pollen Allergies

American Academy of Allergy Asthma and Immunology, http://www.aaaai.org/

Floridata, http://www.floridata.com

Florida 4-H Forest Ecology, http://www.sfrc.ufl.edu/4h/index.html

Florida Automated Weather Network, http://fawn.ifas.ufl.edu/

Florida Fire Weather, http://www.fl-dof.com/fire_weather/index.html

Florida Plants, http://www.floridaplants.com

Florida Allergy Forecast, http://www.pollen.com/state.asp?id=fl

Florida Nature, http://www.floridanature.org/

Florida Natural Areas Inventory, http://www.fnai.org/FieldGuide/search_001.cfm

National Garden Bureau, http://www.ngb.org/

Tom Volk's Fungi, http://tomvolkfungi.net/

University of Florida IFAS Extension, http://edis.ifas.ufl.edu/

USDA Plant Database, http://plants.usda.gov/

Part II. Arthropods

Acari: Mites and Ticks, A Virtual Introduction, http://www.sel.barc.usda.gov/acari/index.html

Arboviral Disease: Florida Department of Health, http://www.myfloridaeh.com/community/arboviral/

Bed bug Registry, http://bedbugregistry.com/

Bees of Florida, http://chiron.valdosta.edu/jbpascar/Intro.htm

Bug Guide.net, http://bugguide.net

BlattaBase: The Cockroach Homepage, http://www.bio.umass.edu/
biology/kunkel/cockroach.html

EPA Bed bug Information, http://epa.gov/bedbugs/

Florida Ants, http://www.antweb.org/florida.jsp

Florida Mosquito Database, http://mosquito.ifas.ufl.edu/FMD/Florida_
Mosquito_Database.html

Household Products Database: Pesticides, http://hpd.nlm.nih.gov/cgi-bin/
household/prodtree?prodcat=Pesticides

Mosquito Information Website, http://mosquito.ifas.ufl.edu/

Smithsonian Institution Bug Info, http://www.si.edu/encyclopedia_si/
nmnh/buginfo/start.htm

USDA Systemic Entomology Laboratory, http://www.ars.usda.gov/Main/
site_main.htm?modecode=12-75-41-00

University of Florida Entomology and Nematology, http://entomology.
ifas.ufl.edu/publicat.html

Venomous Creatures of Florida, http://www.miamipoison.org/x34.xml

Part III. Plant-related Allergies

American Latex Allergy Association, http://www.latexallergyresources.
org/

Botanical Dermatology Online Textbook, http://www.telemedicine.org/
stamford.htm

Center for Aquatic and Invasive Plants, http://plants.ifas.ufl.edu/

Food and Drug Administration, http://www.fda.gov/

Global Invasive Species database, http://www.issg.org/database/welcome/

Invasive Species Index, http://www.invasive.org

Poisonous Plants of Florida, http://www.med.miami.edu/poisoncontrol/
x35.xml

Part IV. Sea Life

Florida Fish and Wildlife Conservation Commission Harmful Algal
Blooms, http://research.myfwc.com/features/view_article.asp?id=9670

Centers for Disease Control Environmental Health, http://www.cdc.gov/
Environmental/

Fish Database, http://fishbase.org

Florida Seafood, http://www.fl-seafood.com
Harmful Algae Page, http://www.whoi.edu/redtide/
Florida Dept. of Health, http://www.myfloridaeh.com/
Florida Seafood, http://www.fl-seafood.com/

Index

Page numbers in *italics* refer to illustrations.

Theresa Willingham is a professional writer with more than 25 years of experience that includes extensive coverage of education, health, family, and environmental issues. Her first book, *The Food Allergy Field Guide: A Lifestyle Manual for Families* (Savory Palate, 2nd ed., 2006), focuses on empowering families and children with food allergies to take charge of their lives. She is a longtime family advocate, supporting with her writing and volunteer efforts the rights of all people to direct their own learning, health, and well-being. She is founder and president of Learning Is for Everyone, Inc., a nationwide nonprofit educational resource organization based in Tampa. She is also lead organizer of Florida's first TEDxYouth program, an independently organized TED event for youth. A lifelong Floridian and avid outdoorsperson, she enjoys canoeing and kayaking, hiking, beachcombing, nature watching and photography, fishing, geocaching with her husband, Steve, and their three mostly grown children, Ellie, Andrea, and Chris, and just generally soaking up Florida's remarkable outdoors!